Breast Cancer Nursing

Breast Cancer Nursing

Edited by
Sylvia Denton

CHAPMAN & HALL

London · Glasgow · Weinheim · New York · Tokyo · Melbourne · Madras

Published by Chapman & Hall, 2–6 Boundary Row, London SE1 8HN, UK

Chapman & Hall, 2–6 Boundary Row, London SE1 8HN, UK

Blackie Academic and Professional, Wester Cleddens Road, Bishopbriggs, Glasgow G64 2NZ, UK

Chapman & Hall GmbH, Pappelallee 3, 69469 Weinheim, Germany

Chapman & Hall USA, 115 Fifth Avenue, 41st Floor, New York NY 10119, USA

Chapman & Hall Japan, ITP-Japan, Kyowa Building, 3F, 2-2-1 Hirakawacho, Chiyoda-ku, Tokyo 102, Japan

Chapman & Hall Australia, 102 Dodds Street, South Melbourne, Victoria 3205, Australia

Chapman & Hall India, R. Seshadri, 32 Second Main Road, CIT East, Madras 600 035, India

First edition 1996
Reprinted 1996

© 1996   Chapman & Hall

This edition not for sale in North America and Australia; orders from these regions should be referred to Singular Publishing Group, Inc., 4284 41st Street, San Diego, CA92105, USA

Typeset in 10/12 Times by Mews Photosetting, Beckenham, Kent
Printed in Great Britain by St Edmundsbury Press Limited, Bury St Edmunds, Suffolk.

ISBN 0 412 41200 4

A catalogue record for this book is available from the British Library

♾ Printed on permanent acid-free text paper, manufactured in accordance with ANSI/NISO Z39.48-1992 and ANSI/NISO Z39.48-1984 (Permanence of Paper).

Contents

Contributors

Caroline Badger
Macmillan Nurse Consultant in Lymphoedema.

Heather Brown
Clinical Nurse Specialist – Breast Care, Royal Berkshire & Battle Hospitals
   NHS Trust, Reading.

Trish Cotton
Senior Nurse, Senior Breast Care Nurse, Cardiff.

Sylvia Denton
Senior Clinical Nurse Specialist – Breast Care, St Bartholomews Hospital,
   London.

Deborah Fenlon
Senior Clinical Nurse Specialist, Breast Care, The Royal Marsden NHS Trust,
   Surrey.

Kate Gowshall
Formerly Senior Clinical Nurse Specialist – Breast Care, Northwick Park
   Hospital NHS Trust, Harrow, Middlesex.

Maureen Hunter
Rehabilitation Services Manager, The Royal Marsden NHS Trust, London.

Gill Oliver
Director of Patient Services, Clatterbridge Centre for Oncology, Bebington,
   Wirral, Merseyside.

Joanna M. Parker
Formerly Clinical Nurse Specialist – Breast Care, Royal Marsden Hospital,
   London.

Clare Shaw
Chief Dietician, The Royal Marsden NHS Trust, London.

Clare Sleigh
Chartered Physiotherapist, West Midlands.

Ann Tait
Macmillan Nurse Researcher, London.

Annie Topping
Senior Lecturer in Nursing/Health Studies, University of Huddersfield, Huddersfield.

Richard Wells
Formerly Rehabilitation Services Manager, Royal Marsden NHS Trust, London & Surrey

Nicky West
Clinical Nurse Specialist – Breast Care, University Hospital of Wales, Cardiff.

Foreword

In recent years, an expanding body of research evidence has begun to high-light the value of nursing care. This evidence confirms what nurses have known for many years – that nursing care helps more patients to get better quicker. Patients value nurses as those members of the health care team that make them feel 'human' and ensure that their treatment is not more of an ordeal than their illness. The research also shows that nursing care is value for money.

For the 29 000 women who are diagnosed with breast cancer annually, the value of nursing is self evident. Every woman should have access to the care, expertise and support of a breast care nurse.

Nursing care is changing. Patients are rightly more informed about different treatment options and more assertive in seeking high quality services. They are much more likely to be aware that breast care nurses have a special service to offer and they are very likely to want help and support at home as well as or instead of in hospital.,

The outreach work of breast care nurses provides a model for many other patient services where people need continuous support from before diagnosis, through diagnosis, surgery or treatment, to after care, rehabilitation and monitoring.

Standard setting work such as that undertaken by the RCN Breast Care Nursing Society, and the National Breast Screening Programme, are helping to ensure that women with breast cancer get the services they want and need and provide models for care delivery for other health problems.

Clearly, nurses bring a new dimension to care, increasing the variety as well as the volume and the quality of care available.

This book reflects nursing's contribution to the care of people with breast cancer. Sylvia Denton has drawn together the excellent research, experience and practice of the authors; nurses who are leading the way in this vital field of health care. A number of them have given their time, commitment and expertise to the RCN.

Thus, the book is an invaluable resource for nurses who are actively involved in breast care and those who want to consolidate and expand their practice to offer greater choice to patients and clients.

As such, *Breast Cancer Nursing* is an excellent working guide and a constructive tool in the care of patients with breast cancer.

Christine Hancock
Royal College of Nursing

Introduction

1

Sylvia Denton

For as long as man has sought to unravel the complexities of human disease, breast cancer has been a subject of study. Hippocrates, considered to be one of the founders of modern medicine, described it some four centuries BC, and those practising in the field of medicine since have added their beliefs about the nature and appropriate treatment for breast cancer to the records.

Today, cancer of the breast is one of the most topical and controversial subjects in oncology, not least because it is so common. Among women it is the most common malignancy and a leading cause of cancer death. The world-wide incidence of breast cancer is increasing (Benson *et al.*, 1993), but varies markedly from country to country. There is a very high incidence in North America and northern Europe, and a low incidence in Asia and parts of Africa. Overall, there is a world average of 65 cases of breast cancer per 100 000 people (Souhami *et al.*, 1987).

These facts alone demonstrate the size of the health problem presented by breast cancer, and the enormity of the challege it sets health care professionals in meeting the needs of and caring for those who have or fear they may have the disease.

One of the most important factors in caring for women with breast cancer is teamwork based on a clear understanding of how the expertise of each member of the multidisciplinary team can contribute to the total care of the individual. Such care must be founded on appropriately informed research-based practice. The King's Fund Forum (1986) has published guidelines for the treatment of primary breast cancer that recommend it be undertaken by a multidisciplinary team with special responsibility for this area of care.

INCIDENCE OF BREAST CANCER

In the UK approximately 29 000 are diagnosed as having breast cancer and 15 000 die from it every year. Breast cancer accounts for 5% of all female deaths and 19% of all new cases of cancer among females. Overall, breast cancer affects 1 in 12 women.

Over the 40-year period 1951–90, mortality rates for women aged 15–44 years showed a slight decrease, but the rate increased in the older age groups (Cancer Research Campaign, 1991). Currently, the five-year relative survival rate of all women diagnosed with breast cancer in England and Wales is 62%.

The standardized mortality rate for breast cancer in England and Wales is 28.4 per 100 000 females, which makes the UK the world leader for mortality from breast cancer. The government has set a target for the reduction of breast cancer mortality in the UK by 25% in women aged 50–65 years by the year 2000, largely through the implementation of the National Breast Screening Programme (The Health of the Nation, 1992).

AETIOLOGY

Epidemiological factors demonstrate that breast cancer is a heterogeneous disease and every woman is randomly at risk of developing it at some time in her life. However, there are a number of risk factors that appear to increase the probability of a woman developing breast cancer.

Studies have shown that endocrine factors play an important role in the development of breast cancer and a number of the risk factors identified relate to a woman's reproductive history: an early menarche, a late menopause, nulliparity and late child bearing (first child after 30 years of age) are all considered to contribute to a higher risk of breast cancer (Miller and Bulbrook, 1980).

A family history of breast cancer is another factor that has been identified as increasing risk. This factor is particularly significant if a first degree relative (i.e. a mother, sister or daughter) was pre-menopausal at the time of her diagnosis. Other risk factors are increasing age and obesity. Factors thought to increase risk but yet to be fully evaluated are a high fat diet, high doses of hormone replacement therapy for a prolonged period of time and the prolonged use of combined oral contraceptives at a very early age or prior to the first pregnancy.

It is important, especially for those caring for patients, to maintain a sense of perspective with regard to risk factors and to consider the anxiety and guilt such information may engender, particularly as the majority of such factors are beyond an individual's control. It is especially important to bear this in mind when talking to patients and their families about hereditary risk factors.

Genetic factors in breast cancer are currently receiving a great deal of attention, but the identifiction of predisposing genes for breast cancer has practical implications for those identified as having an inherited risk of contracting the disease and these must be addressed as research programmes develop.

GENETIC FACTORS IN BREAST CANCER
Heather Brown

A somatic cell contains a nucleus within which are two sets of chromosomes. Members of each identical pair are called 'homologues'. Cells multiply and divide in two ways:

- **Mitosis** is the process of cell division whereby the cell and nucleus divide in two, and each duplicated chromosome also divides in two, thus making the same number of chromosomes in the nucleus of the newly formed cell.
- **Meiosis** is the process of nuclear division involving the formation of gametes, where the number of chromosomes is halved. Each mature gamete contains one chromatid from one of the pair of homologous chromosomes (thus the diploid number becomes halved or haploid). At fertilization, when the zygote is formed, the cell once again has the full number of chromosomes.

In the normal human there are two sets of 23 single chromosomes, one set of 23 from the father and one set of 23 from the mother. Twenty-two of these pairs are 'identical' (autosomal), the remaining pair, the sex chromosomes, differ for males or females. The female chromosomes are typed 'XX' and the male ones as 'XY'.

Chromosomes contain genes, or characteristics. The chromosomes, but not the genes within, can actually be seen through a microscope, especially during cell division.

Genes are large molecules made up of deoxyribonucleic acid (DNA) whose double helical structure allows both copying and division. The threadlike substance of DNA consists of millions and millions of chemical bases: adenine, guanine (purines), thymine and cytosine (pyrimidines). The nucleotide bases can only bond in specific pairs, adenine with thymine and guanine with cytosine. The two antiparallel strands twist around each other to form a double helix. These are organised in a consistent and specific pattern along the chromosome, resulting in an almost universal gene complement. There are over 50 000 genes located on the human chromosomes.

Along the length of a chromosome is a single centromere, which effects the division of the chromosome into two arms. The shorter arm is designated **p** (for petit) and the longer arm is known as **q** (Figure 1.1).

Genes along a chromosome may be dominant or recessive. In the former situation, a single allele will result in a predictable phenotype. If a gene is truly dominant, then the phenotype should be independent of whether it is present as a single copy (Aa), i.e. heterozygous, or as two copies (AA), i.e. homozygous state. By comparison, a recessive gene will usually only result in a recognisable phenotype when present in the homozygous state (aa).

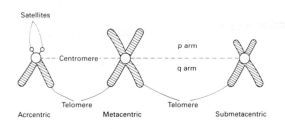

Figure 1.1 The anatomy of the human chromosome.

The particular sequence of individual chemical sub-units in a gene serves as a molecular code to specify the manufacture of a particular protein; an alteration (mutation) at even a single position of the DNA sequence may cause serious malfunction of the resulting protein.

The p53 protein is a product of a nuclear oncogene and appears to be responsible for preventing cellular division in an uncontrolled fashion. As such, it works by stabilizing the cell, and abnormalities might, therefore, be expected to allow uncontrolled growth. The protein occurs both as a wild type and as a mutant. It now seems that an abnormality in the p53 expression is associated with an increased risk of numerous tumours, including clusters of breast cancer sarcomas, adrenocortical carcinomas, leukaemias and brain tumours (the Li-Fraumeni syndrome) (Dixon and Sainsbury, 1993).

Recent research has shown that at least three, probably five or more, genes are implicated in familial breast cancer. The BRCA1 gene is located on the long arm of chromosome 17 (namely 17q 12–21), and P53, the tumour suppressor gene, is located on the short arm of chromosome 17 (17p). The BRCA1 gene was cloned in 1994 (Miki *et al.*, 1994) and together with the loss of the nm23 anti-metastatic gene, was suspected to be involved in sporadic breast cancer (Wallace, 1993). However, preliminary data (Futreal *et al.*, 1994; Boyd, 1995) suggest that causative mutations in BRCA1, in sporadic breast cancers, may be rare. At the same time that the cloning of BRCA1 was described, Wooster *et al.* (1994) reported the localization of a second gene, BRCA2, on the long arm of chromosome 13. Mutations of this gene are also associated with a high risk of breast cancer, but are rarely implicated in ovarian cancer.

Inherited risk of breast cancer

Family history is recognized as an important, identifiable risk factor for breast cancer, albeit for only a small percentage of women (Sibbering *et al.*, 1993);

it has an age incidence curve shifted towards early onset disease. It has also been suggested that the familial form of breast malignancy may result in significantly improved survival than for breast cancer as a whole (Porter *et al.*, 1993).

It now seems fairly conclusive that only about 4–5% of breast cancers are due to the highly penetrant dominant gene (Evans *et al.*, 1994). When breast cancer is hereditary, 40% of those families demonstrate a mutation on the BRCA1 gene (Dixon and Sainsbury, 1993) and approximately 35% of the remainder on the BRCA2 gene. The earlier a breast cancer presents, the greater the likelihood of an inherited aetiology (Claus, Risch and Thompson, 1990). Obviously this risk also increases the higher the number of affected relatives (especially first degree relatives), with bilateral breast cancer and with a history of related cancers (Claus, Risch and Thompson, 1990; Easton *et al.*, 1993; Evans *et al.*, 1994).

Practical implications

'Family cancer clinics' have now been set up in most regions for patients considered to be at a high risk of developing breast cancer through familial traits. These clinics offer risk assessment, screening and counselling for the women and their families (Easton *et al.*, 1993).

Having identified an 'at risk' woman, what help is available? Clinical breast examination is usually offered as well as mammographic screening, either annually or biennially. An extreme form of management for those considered to be at very high risk of developing breast cancer is to perform bilateral subcutaneous mastectomy or simple mastectomy; this is currently very rarely employed in the UK. Trials of 'preventive agents', such as Tamoxifen, are also currently underway.

Meanwhile, the ethical and legal implications of developments such as genetic testing for breast cancer must be monitored and considered. How should women be informed of the potential and limitations of genetic testing? How should pre- and post-test counselling services be established? And, most importantly, what are the long-term effects on the individual and the family?

The high level of interest breast cancer generally attracts suggests that there could be great demand for genetic testing for it. Even if such demand is confined to those women who have increased risk because of family history, it could still involve tens of thousands of women, and the practical implications of this one service have to be considered in parallel with scientific development. Moreover, the apparent low percentage of familial cases and mutations in BRCA1 in sporadic breast cancer probably indicates that mutation studies will have less benefit or impact on the general population.

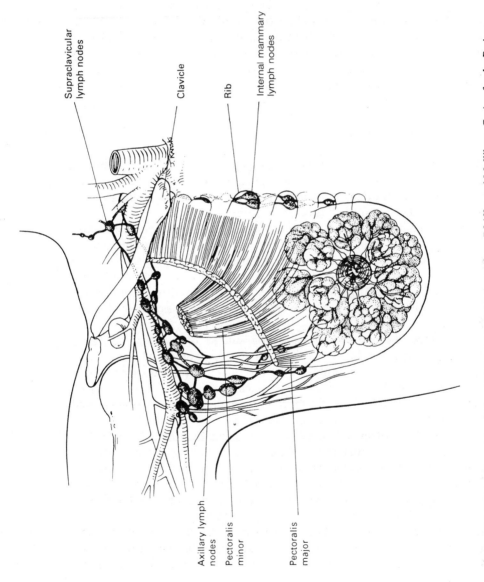

Figure 1.2 Schematic representation of the breast. Reproduced from Pfeiffer and Mulliken, *Caring for the Patient with Breast Cancer*, published by Reston Publishing Co., 1984.

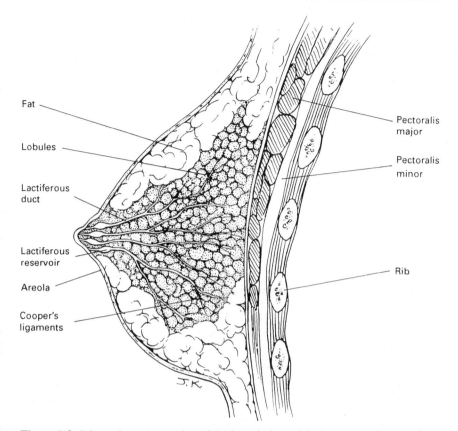

Fat

Lobules

Lactiferous duct

Lactiferous reservoir

Areola

Cooper's ligaments

Pectoralis major

Pectoralis minor

Rib

Figure 1.3 Schematic representation of the lateral view of the breast. Reproduced from Pfeiffer and Mulliken, *Caring for the Patient with Breast Cancer*, published by Reston Publishing Co., 1984.

STRUCTURE AND FUNCTION OF THE FEMALE BREAST

As with all anatomy the structure of the female breast is related to its function; prior to discussing histological diagnosis of disease and treatment options, it seems pertinent to consider its structure and function.

The breast is considered to be a modified sweat gland that rests on the anterior rib-cage. The breast disc extends superiorly to the clavicle, medially to the sternum, laterally to the latissimus dorsi muscle and inferiorly to the costal margin (Figure 1.2). The function of this organ is to produce a supply of nourishment for the new-born baby, initially colostrum and within a few days milk.

The breast tissue consists of between 15 and 20 glandular milk-producing units arranged radially around the nipple, each consisting of lobular units or alveoli. The milk is produced by the epithelial cell lining of the alveoli and is secreted into the lumen of the gland. Clusters of alveoli supply the small lactiferous ducts that unite with other ducts to form one large excretory duct for each system. These ducts enlarge into reservoirs and then constrict and converge together to empty out at the nipple (Figure 1.3). The glandular units are surrounded by two layers of fibrous tissue joining the two suspensory ligaments (Cooper's liagments) and fatty adipose tissue.

The nipple contains small muscle fibres that react to stimulation and temperature. The areola has very small glands that expand during pregnancy to boost the milk supply. The breast tissue is contained within overlaying layers of subcutaneous fat and skin.

The lymphatic system within the breast is extensive and drains in several directions, mainly to regional lymph nodes in the axilla but also via nodes in the supraclavicular region and in the internal mammary chain.

As a sexual organ the breast is directly controlled by hormones, predominantly those from the pituitary gland and the ovaries. During each menstrual cycle the breasts undergo changes associated with blood concentrations of the hormones oestrogen and progesterone.

The breast is a highly vascular organ, well served by a good arterial blood supply and venous drainage. The two main arteries are the axillary artery and the internal mammary artery.

Four main muscles are associated with the breast. Immediately under the breast is the pectoralis major muscle; it is triangular in shape, stretching from the clavicle to the sternum, to the 6th and 7th ribs and the humerus. Underlying this is the smaller pectoralis minor muscle, stretching from the 3rd, 4th and 5th ribs to the scapula. The serratus anterior muscle arises from the ribs at the side of the chest to the scapula. The latissimus dorsi muscle goes from the spine to the humerus at the back of the axilla.

PATHOLOGY

Various procedures may be undertaken in order to reach a diagnosis of breast cancer, but the final diagnosis depends on cytological or histological evaluation (Carlson, 1991). Histological evaluation can provide important prognostic information as well as final diagnosis.

The two major criteria used in the classification of breast cancer are the cell type of the tumour and whether the tumour is contained within the duct system – is it *in situ* or has it invaded outside the basement cell membrane into the stroma of the breast? Millis (1983) states that carcinoma is *in situ* when the malignant cellular change is restricted to the epithelial surface.

There are different histopathological types of breast cancer, but the majority of primary breast cancers are found to be adenocarcinomas arising from the epithelial lining of the terminal duct lobular unit. Infiltrating ductal carcinoma is the most frequent and accounts for 75% of breast cancers (Stuart Goodman, 1987).

Hitherto, *in situ* breast cancers accounted for about 7% of the total breast cancers detected (Millis, 1983) – often presenting as a blood-stained nipple discharge or a lump – but the number of women diagnosed with *in situ* disease has increased considerably since the introduction of the National Breast Screening Programme in the UK since mammography identifies the calcification frequently found in ductal *carcinoma in situ* (DCIS) (Vessey, 1991). Breast screening centres have seen a three- to four-fold rise in the incidence of DCIS (Cooke, 1989) since commencement of The National Health Service Breast Screening Programme. Other tumour types frequently encountered are lobular carcinoma (which is frequently bilateral) mucoid carcinoma, tubular carcinoma and medullary carcinoma.

Paget's disease of the nipple and inflammatory breast cancer both have particular clinical characteristics. Paget's disease of the nipple manifests itself by producing an 'eczematous' type of eruption on or around the nipple. This may occur together with *in situ* or infiltrating duct carcinoma (Millis, 1983). Inflammatory breast cancer is a poorly differentiated ductal carcinoma showing erythema of the skin and often involving a large area of the breast. It is an aggressive form of disease with extensive local involvement of the dermal lymphatics.

The grading of the tumour is important in the pathological assessment of tumours as it may be predictive of how aggressive the cancer is, and thus reflect prognosis. Low-grade tumours tend to resemble the original normal cell, whereas tumour cells of a higher grade appear unlike the normal cell and may represent a more aggressive type of disease.

Other tumours in the breast of connective tissue origin, for example sarcoma, are rare, as is metastatic spread to the breast from cancer elsewhere in the body.

STAGING

Once a diagnosis of breast cancer has been established, the staging of the disease provides the basis for the selection of the appropriate treatment to manage both

Table 1.1 TNM staging in breast cancer*

TO	No palpable tumour
T1[+]	Tumour 2 cm or less in diameter
T2[+]	Tumour 2–5 cm in diameter
T3[+]	Tumour > 5 cm
T4	Tumour of any size with fixation to chest wall or skin
NO	No palpable node involvement
N1	Mobile ipsilateral nodes
N2	Fixed ipsilateral nodes
N3	Supraclavicular or infraclavicular nodes, or oedema of arm
MO	No distant metastases
M1	Distant metastases

*Source: the International Union Against Cancer.
[+] Suffix 'a' with T1–T3 denotes no fixation of the tumour to underlying pectoral facia or muscle. Suffix 'b' denotes fixation.

Table 1.2 Combination of the TNM classifications*

Stage I	Small tumour (<2 cm)
Stage II	Tumour >2 cm but <5 cm, lymph nodes negative or Tumour <5 cm, lymph nodes positive, no detectable distant metastases
Stage III	Large tumour (>5 cm) or Tumour of any size with invasion of skin or chest wall or Associated with positive lymph nodes in the supra/clavicular region, but no detectable distant metastases
Stage IV	Tumour of any size Lymph nodes either positive or negative Distant metastases

*Source: the International Union Against Cancer.

the local disease within the breast and the potential/existing metastasis. Staging demonstrates the known extent of the disease at that time.

The TNM (tumour node metastasis) staging system, as outlined by the International Union Against Cancer (Table 1.1), is widely-used to classify breast cancer. Combinations of the TNM configuration are used to define clinical staging (Table 1.2).

ADVANCED DISEASE

A proportion of patients who have undergone treatment for early breast cancer experience a recurrence in the form of metastatic disease; some patients have this diagnosed when they first attend hospital. The nature of breast cancer is such that the first recurrence of disease may occur many years after the initial diagnosis.

In a large study conducted by Brinkley and Haybittle (1975), the overall reported survival rate of patients was 20% after 25 years. For women who had initially been diagnosed with 'early' breast cancer, i.e. stage I and II disease, the 25-year survival rate was 30%. The five-year relative survival rate for women presenting with metastatic breast cancer, i.e. stage IV disease, is 18% (CRC, 1991).

The four main areas that have the potential for metastatic spread from the breast are the bones, lungs, liver and brain. It is generally considered that the treatments currently available do not provide a cure for metastatic breast cancer (Aisner, 1983; Carlson, 1991; Howell and Ribeiro, 1985). However, control of disease and palliation of symptoms in order to achieve a good quality of life is, for many, a legitimate goal. Howell states (Howell and Ribeiro, 1985):

Patients will spend a considerable period of time with overt disease, this is not a time for nihilism but more for quiet optimism ... With good general care the quality of life can usually be maintained until very near the end of life.

The treatments employed to treat breast cancer at all stages of disease are discussed in the following chapters. However, it should be noted that women experiencing recurrent or metastatic disease frequently require very concentrated care with regular follow-up. These women are likely to relive much of the trauma they experienced at initial diagnosis, but with more intensity; there is often a feeling of 'being let down' and acute disappointment, which may lead to clinically significant anxiety and/or depression. Pinder and co-workers (1993) reported that in a study of psychiatric illness among a group of 139 women with advanced breast cancer, 25% of the women were experiencing clinical states of anxiety and/or depression. These levels of psychiatric disorder are equal to those experienced after inital diagnosis.

If the woman was involved in treatment choice at the initial diagnosis she may have feelings of doubt and, indeed, guilt at a recurrence. The opportunity to discuss such feelings should be given, and emotional support and information may be necessary if she needs to undergo further diagnostic investigations and is once again invited to participate in selecting a treatment option.

In particular, the woman must be reassured that her carers will not abandon her as she once again faces a further diagnosis of cancer. Patients often ask 'Is it hopeless?' Such a question must be answered not only with honesty, but also with sensitivity and the maintenance of hope: patients are often more afraid of pain than they are of the progression of their illness.

At this stage of the disease it is often very important to review a patient's understanding of her situation and discover if there is any further information she requires. Again, this should be given with sensitivity and without invading personal privacy. Not only might the woman require an ever-increasing degree of emotional and practical support, she may well be trying to come to terms with the fact of her own mortality. Patients often express feelings of loneliness, even though surrounded by relatives, friends and professionals.

At this stage of the disease patients frequently find any treatment particularly exhausting. Review of the treatment and its side-effects, and consideration of how these might be managed and life 'paced' may help the patient to anticipate problems before she encounters them and thus to gain confidence and encouragement and, above all, to feel in control. Care must be taken to meet the patient's need for information, practical help and emotional support, and to express her sexuality and spirituality during this time.

MALE BREAST CANCER

Although rare, breast cancer can affect men: approximately 200 men a year develop breast cancer in the UK, and 90 men a year die from it; 1% of all breast cancers affect men, usually at an older age than women. Those affected often undergo surgery for primary breast cancer, and the treatments offered are generally similar to those for female breast cancer. Patterson, Battersby and Bach (1980) reported that when tamoxifen was given to men with breast cancer it produced a remission in nearly half of those treated.

Because it is such a rare condition, little has been recorded about the psychosocial problems encountered by men with breast cancer. The man must cope initially with the rarity of his illness, which could make him feel isolated and embarrassed, especially as he has to come to terms with a disease that is predominantly female.

Treatment may necessitate castration, which can profoundly affect a man's body image. In addition, as in women, men may develop lymphoedema of the upper limb, which can be incapacitating as well as being a constant reminder for the patient of the disease. The man with breast cancer needs the same care as a woman, plus an understanding of his special requirements as a man with this disease.

CONCLUSION

Those who care for patients with breast cancer must understand the natural history, diagnosis and treatment of this complex disease, and the controversies that frequently surround its management. However, just as important, is an understanding of the type of care and support that patients need as they respond to the diagnosis and treatment of breast cancer. That care should be the result of activities and an environment that make people feel valued and safe, minimizing both physiological and psychological distress while promoting independence for the patient.

Roach (1984) identified five attributes of caring: compassion, competence, conscience, commitment and confidence. If applying these to the care of patients with breast cancer they could be interpreted thus:

- Compassion is being with and experiencing with the patient but not expressing pity; it might be described as empathy. 'To be alongside' the patient, demonstrating support but maintaining patient dignity, is an important concept in cancer care.
- Competence is the knowledge and skills essential to safe care and practice.
- The concept of conscience emphasizes the need to maintain independence of choice for the patient and respect for the individual as a whole.
- Commitment emphasizes the quality of investment of those who care and undertake the task in hand.
- Confidence is that which fosters trusting relationships, is an aid to the delivery of information and gives the patient the feeling of social support.

Care is not unique to any one discipline, Tschudin (1986) states:

The subject of caring is never exhausted. Each day we meet new different aspects. Caring is a basic human need and a basic primal response to need and as such it always takes place within a relationship. This forms a basis for ethics.

Integrating such concepts into all aspects of the delivery of services and treatment to those with breast cancer could provide the foundation for care of the highest order.

REFERENCES

Aisner, J. (1983) Chemotherapy in the treatment for Advanced Breast Cancer, in *Contemporary Issues in Clinical Oncology – Breast Cancer* (ed. R. Margolese), Churchill Livingstone, New York.

Benson, J.R., Lau, Y., Jatoi, I. and Baum, M. (1993) Early breast cancer: diagnosis and management. *Postgraduate Update*, 15 September, 337–43.

Boyd, J. (1995) BRCA1: More than a hereditary breast cancer gene? *Nature Genetics*, **9**, 335-6.

Brinkley, D. and Haybittle, J.L. (1975) The curability of breast cancer, *Lancet*, ii, 95–7.

Cancer Research Campaign (CRC) (1991) *Breast Cancer Fact Sheet 6.2*, Cancer Research Campaign, London.

Carlson, J. (1991) Breast cancer, in *Oncology Nursing* (ed. S.E. Otto), Mosby, Missouri, MO.

Claus, E.B., Risch, N.J. and Thompson, W.D. (1990) Age at onset of familial breast cancer. *American Journal of Epidemiology*, 131, 961–72.

Cooke, T.G. (1989) Ductal carcinoma *in situ*; a new clinical problem. *British Journal of Surgery*, **76**, July, 660–2.

Dixon, M. and Sainsbury, R. (1993) *Handbook of Diseases of the Breast*, Churchill Livingstone, Edinburgh.

Easton, D.F., Bishop, D.T., Ford, D., Crockford, G.P. (1993) The Breast Cancer Linkage Consortium, Genetic linkage analysis in familial breast and ovarian cancer: results from 214 families. *American Journal of Human Genetics*, **52**, 678–701.

Evans, D.G.R., Fentiman, I.S., McPherson, K. *et al.* (1994) Familial breast cancer. *British Medical Journal*, **308**, 183–7.

Futreal, P.A., Liu, Q., Shattuck-Eidens, D., Cochran, C., Harshman, K. *et al.* (1994) BRCA1 mutations in primary breast and ovarian carcinomas. *Science*, **266**, 120–22.

Howell, A. and Ribeiro, G. (1985) Management of advanced carcinoma of the breast. *The Practitioner*, **229**, March, 255–62.

King's Fund Forum (1986) Consensus development conference, treatment of primary breast cancer. *British Medical Journal*, **293**, 946–7.

Marshall, E. (1993) Search for a killer: focus shifts from fat to hormones. *Science*, **259**, 618–21.

Miki, Y., Swensen, J., Shattuck-Eidens, D., Futreal, P.A., Harshman, K. *et al.* (1994) A strong candidate for the breast and ovarian cancer susceptibility gene BRCA1. *Science*, **266**, 66–71.

Miller, A.B. and Bulbrook, R.D. (1980) The epidemiology and aetiology of breast cancer, *New England Journal of Medicine*, **303**, 1246–8.

Millis, R. (1983) Principles of Breast Pathology, in *Diagnosis of Breast Disease* (ed. C.A. Parsons), Chapman & Hall, London, pp. 26–53.

Patterson, J.S., Battersby, L.A. and Bach, B.K. (1980) Use of tamoxifen in advanced male breast cancer. *Cancer Treatment Reports*, **64**, 801–4.

Pinder, K.L., Ramirez, A.J., Black, M.E. *et al.* (1993) Psychiatric disorder in patients with advanced breast cancer: prevalence and associated factors, *European Journal of Cancer*, **29A**(4), 524–7.

Porter, D.E., Chetty, U., Dixon, J.M. and Steel, C.M. (1993) Breast cancer in the BRCA1 gene carriers results in significantly better survival than in sporadic breast cancer. *The Breast*, **2**, 187.

Roach, M.S. (1984) *The Human Mode of Being, Implications for Nursing*, Faculty of Nursing, University of Toronto, Toronto.

Sibbering, D.M., Holland, P., Mitchell, A.K. and Blamey, R.W. (1993) Screening the at risk patient: family history. *The Breast*, **2**, 186.

Souhami, R., Tobias, J. (1987) *Cancer and its management*, Blackwell Scientific Publications, Oxford.

Stuart Goodman, M. (1987) Breast Malignancies, in *Cancer Nursing Principles and Practice*, Jones and Bartlett, Boston.

The Health of the Nation – a strategy for health in England (1992), HMSO, London.

Tschudin, V. (1986) *Ethics in Nursing*, Heinemann, London.

Vessey, M. (1991) *Breast Cancer Screening 1991: Evidence and Experience Since the Forrest Report*, NHS BSP publication.

Wallace, M., Thompson, A.M., Cohen, B. *et al.* (1993) Evidence for involvement of the breast cancer 1 (BRC A1) gene in sporadic breast cancer. *The Breast*, **2**, 187.

Wooster, R., Neuhausen, S.L., Mangion, J., Quirk, Y., Ford, D. *et al.* (1994) Localization of a breast cancer susceptibility gene, BRCA2, to chromosome 13q 12–13. *Science*, **265**, 2088–90.

Psychological aspects of breast cancer

2

Ann Tait

INTRODUCTION

The psychosocial and ethical aspects of patient care are of great importance when nursing women who have, or fear they have, breast cancer. It is a particularly emotive subject and has come to be seen as an important topic by the media: breast cancer makes 'good' headlines. Unfortunately, reports on breast cancer issues are sometimes presented in a 'sensationalized' way and thus contribute to the psychosocial problems faced by patients and those who seek to care for them.

However, one potentially positive outcome of all the publicity given to breast cancer over the past decade has been a considerable increase in awareness, among the public and health care professionals alike, of the emotional problems related to this disease. This can be attributed not just to the media but also to the professional dissemination of research findings and the practical work of various organizations, charitable or otherwise, that give information and support at national and local level.

One result of this increased interest and knowledge is that there is a growing recognition of the need to provide adequate care. It is now accepted that breast cancer nurses should be integral members of the specialist team (Cancer Relief Macmillan Fund, 1994) and that nursing care should include adequate psychosocial assessment of individual need, followed by the giving of appropriate information, practical help, emotional support and, where necessary, referral to other agencies. This can improve the quality of life of a patient with breast cancer, even when medical treatment may be unsuccessful (Cotton *et al.*, 1991, Maguire *et al.*, 1980a; RCN, 1994; Maguire, 1994; Watson *et al.*, 1988; Wilkinson, Maguire and Tait, 1988).

Anderson (1988) outlined the rehabilitative role of the nurse as patient educator, counsellor and co-ordinator. As the number of patients surviving for longer periods increases, nurses can contribute to the quality and satisfaction of patients' lives by developing rehabilitation principles as an integral part of their practice, she says. Such care can be challenging and difficult, but it can also be rewarding.

PROBLEMS FACED BY PATIENTS

Threat of mortality

For most patients, the overriding concern is the threat to life (Denton and Baum, 1982; Fallowfield *et al.*, 1990); even the word 'cancer' is often equated with death. And when knowledge of treatments precedes knowledge of the aetiology of a disease such as breast cancer, the disease can be perceived as frightening and mysterious (Sontag, 1979).

Many women say that their first thought on realizing they had breast cancer is that they were likely to die. Such fears cannot easily be assuaged for, although many women with breast cancer die from other causes, it is a fact that 16 000 will eventually die from the disease itself in the UK. Until the advent of AIDS, cancer had been unique in the deep-rooted existential fear it provoked, often of a painful and lingering death (Weisman, 1979).

Threat to the breast

Even before treatment, a patient may experience feelings that the breast is damaged because of the stigma of cancer (see below). The threat to the integrity of the breast will vary according to the cosmetic outcome, and the amount and type of surgery or radiation, but, importantly, the perceived threat will vary according to the significance of the breast for each particular woman (Bard and Sutherland, 1952). Although the breast may well be of great sexual significance, women can also consider their breasts to be a necessary part of feeling intrinsically complete as a person, they may feel the need for this sense of completeness as a mother, too.

It is difficult for people with breast cancer to forget about it when the breast and the female form are used so widely in advertising and the media. The pressures to conform to the stereotype are strong, and the more general acceptance of women being free to go 'bra-less' and 'topless' makes it harder for women to cope after treatment.

Other body image pressures may be even stronger, however. In a study comparing self-concept and social function in women with a variety of non-cancer as well as cancer problems, Penman and co-workers (1987) found the most important predictor of body image dissatisfaction in women with breast cancer was being overweight, followed by concerns about lack of social support, concurrent medical problems and low scores on locus of control. And in a study of women's concerns (Fallowfield *et al.*, 1990), only 12% gave breast loss as their primary concern. Similarly, in Denton and Baum's study (1982), only 19 out of 79 patients with early breast cancer gave breast loss as their primary concern.

Chronic uncertainty and constant reminders

Given the known facts and figures on mortality rates from breast cancer (Chapter 1), it is not surprising that some patients and their families have great difficulty adjusting to a lifetime of chronic uncertainty about their prognosis. There is, however, a growing interest in the particular difficulties of 'survivorship' and what can be done to alleviate them (McCaffrey, 1991).

Fears about survival are not helped by the frequent attention paid to breast cancer by the media, especially if a well-known person has a recurrence of, or dies from it, or if questions are raised about the efficacy of particular treatments and the ways they are managed (Badwe *et al.*, 1991; Bagenal *et al.*, 1990; Fentiman and Mansel, 1991).

As members of the public become better informed about breast cancer they may also become more aware that even apparently 'early' disease has probably been present for several years and disseminated by the time it is diagnosed. Reassurances that 'all is well' are unlikely to be believed. Following diagnosis and treatment, any subsequent aches or pains can cause anxiety, with the patient constantly aware that they may herald a recurrence.

Breast cancer patients and those involved with them have no definite proof that any particular measures will reduce or control it, unlike with some other serious diseases. They may be aware of the view held by some researchers that certain psychological attitudes in patients such as accepting the diagnosis with a fighting spirit and being actively involved in their own care (Greer, 1990), could affect the course of their disease; they may then feel guilty if they are unable to behave in this way, thinking they are jeopardizing their chances. Such dilemmas can make it difficult to have any sense of control over what is going on.

Stigma

Theories about the causes of cancer often give patients a sense of guilt and of having been stigmatized. Some wonder if they are somehow responsible for bringing this dreaded disease on themselves. Knopf (1974) found that theories about causation were sometimes related to moral wrongdoing. Patients may also be affected by strong cultural taboos that colour people's perception of the onset of cancer. Patients may blame stressful life events or perhaps their own particular personality type for having caused the disease, despite the lack of definitive evidence to support this notion. In fact, the occurrence of breast cancer cannot, as yet, be blamed on the patient's behaviour, unlike lung cancer, for instance, which may be causally related to smoking.

Diagnosis

The time between discovery of a symptom and the confirmation of a diagnosis of breast cancer is the most anxious time for the great majority of people (Maguire, 1976). The shock of diagnosis can be very great because breast cancer is usually detected in someone who is otherwise well. It can be especially traumatic if that person has not previously been aware of any symptoms, for example if the diagnosis arose as a result of a routine screening (Chapter 4). Those suffering from breast cancer, and sometimes those closest to them, may therefore be under an unusually severe form of stress.

However, in one study (Peters-Golden, 1982), while 59% of healthy men and 26% of healthy women thought that breast cancer was 'the worst thing that can happen to a woman', only 6% of patients thought this. Perhaps this demonstrates the ability of many women to cope with the disease and to manage their worries eventually.

Treatments

All the medical treatments for breast cancer can cause adverse side effects to a greater or lesser extent (Chapters 5, 6, 7 and 8), so their prescription can cause much anxiety and stress. The incidence of anxiety, depression and sexual difficulties increase markedly when toxic regimes of adjuvant chemotherapy are used (Hughson *et al.*, 1987; Maguire *et al.*, 1980b). Steroids are sometimes used for advanced disease and they can induce depression and anxiety, as can radiotherapy (Lucas, Maguire and Reason, 1987; Peck and Boland, 1977).

Lack of consensus about treatments

Perhaps one of the greatest challenges that patients with breast cancer and those who care for them have to face is that there is little real consensus in medical circles about what the optimum treatments should be. In one study, cited at the Consensus Development Conference on the treatment of primary breast cancer (1986), 62 doctors were given two hypothetical women cases and asked to produce a treatment plan for each; a total of 36 different proposals were presented for one woman and 42 for the other.

Because there is no evidence that conservative surgery is more or less effective than a mastectomy in prolonging life, there is now an increasing emphasis on giving patients a choice about surgical treatment. This can exert its own pressures on the patient, her family and the health care providers, especially in the prevailing purchaser/provider-oriented health service.

Although some research findings suggest that many patients can cope with choice (Cotton *et al.*, 1991; Morris and Royle, 1978; Wilson, Heart and Dawes, 1988), Degner and Sloan (1992) and Beaver *et al* (1994) found that a small majority of cancer patients wanted doctors to decide. Another study (Fallowfield *et al.*, 1990) found that patients who were informed about choices in surgical treatment for their primary disease, and who in some cases were able to choose, were less depressed in the year following their surgery than patients who were not given choices.

MEDICAL AND MALE ASSUMPTIONS ABOUT THE PROBLEMS WOMEN MAY FACE

Medical researchers have traditionally assumed that the psychological problems experienced by women after treatment fell into two main categories: the threat to mortality and the threat to the breast. However, the insights of Quint (1964), Rosser (1981) and Morris (1983) showed that in the women's experience these two threats were inextricably linked; because the causes and the course of each individual breast cancer were unknown, and the benefits of subsequent treatment had not been universally proven, a patient's feelings of anxiety and helplessness were not simply related to 'mortality' or 'the breast'.

These three studies also revealed a fundamental unease about the state of medical knowledge about women's experiences, breast cancer and the profession's ability to define and treat it. Morris (1983) stated: 'It is without question men who determine the treatments avilable to women with breast cancer' and went on to question the assumptions that clinicians, who are usually men, often make about how women may feel.

Some of the most powerful insights into how women experience breast cancer come from those who have had the disease and who ask to be understood on their own terms rather than within medical (and sometimes nursing) orthodoxy.

Prior (1987) questioned the way in which her surgeon broke the news of her impending mastectomy, and his assumption that it was not the end of the world because he could make her another breast and that was what he would have wanted for his wife. Spence (1986) writes: 'Given that women are expected to be the object of the male gaze, are expected to beautify themselves in order to become lovable and are still fighting for basic rights over their own bodies, it seemed to me that the breast could be seen as a metaphor for our struggles'. Lorde (1980) similarly questioned the conventional health care emphasis on looking good and feeling happy. 'We are equally destroyed by false happiness and false breasts are the passive acceptance of false values'.

COMPLEMENTARY THERAPIES

Some women have advocated holistic therapies, sometimes in addition to conventional treatment, sometimes as an alternative. Brohn (1987), describing the work of a holistic therapy centre, felt that it offered a sense of wholeness and joy with the possibility that people could be healed in a spiritual sense, whether or not they got rid of the disease. The power of positive thought, allowing patients the opportunity to experience their situation in a different way, is also advocated by Clyne (1989).

Patients and nurses show considerable interest in and commitment to complementary therapies generally and the improved quality of life that patients feel they offer. Such therapies are gaining acceptance in many health care settings from health care professionals; nurses, for example, are increasingly seeking training in a variety of therapies such as relaxation, visualization, massage, reflexology and aromatherapy.

LACK OF SPECIALIST TREATMENT

There is increasing discussion in the media about where patients with breast cancer are best treated and who is best equipped to treat them. As early as 1986, the Consensus Development Conference recommended that there be a specialist multidisciplinary breast team in every health district and that each team should incorporate a suitably trained nurse.

There is growing pressure for patients to be treated by specialist teams, whose members are deemed the most likely to be aware of the latest findings and techniques (Department of Health, 1994). There is also demand for suitable support services to be made available and for there to be at least one breast care nurse in every health district (House of Commons, 1991). However, as yet there are not sufficient resources within the NHS to fund these proposals.

An awareness of such debates can increase the anxiety felt by a patient and her family despite the fact that she may be receiving informed and up to date care in other than specialist centres. Sometimes patients and those working in specialist teams may even devalue the support and care their GP (general practitioner) or community nurse might give, and so miss out on an important source of help.

POST-TREATMENT

This is generally considered to be a stressful time for many patients (Fallowfield, 1991). When what is hopefully life-saving treatment stops, the support of those who administer treatment may also stop. This can make many patients feel especially isolated and fearful as they face the unknown and try to pick up the threads of everyday life. The amount of social support a patient perceives that she has is of great importance in her recovery (Bloom, 1982; Miller and Nygren, 1978; Welch-McCaffrey, 1985).

Patients can feel vulnerable and exposed to scrutiny, and they may worry about what other people will think of them; they may, for example, feel threatened by the private examination of partners when making love. The resumption of valued relationships may prove to be particularly poignant by bringing home the possibility that they may end if the cancer spreads. Return to work may be traumatic (Maguire *et al.*, 1978; Morris, Greer and White, 1977). Some fail to return to work, and the proportion may be as high as 46% if no counselling is given (Maguire and Sellwood, 1982).

RECURRENCE

Not surprisingly, psychological morbidity has been shown to be high in women with advanced disease (Halleral, 1994; Hopwood, 1984; Plumb and Holland, 1981; Silberfarb, Maurer and Crouthameal, 1980). It can be a shattering blow to a patient to find that all the effort, skill and courage used to cope with the primary disease has not been effective in stopping the disease spreading. Such devastating news can also be very upsetting and disheartening for those involved in the care. However, some women experience a strange sense of relief: they had always been anxious the cancer would return and the diagnosis of recurrence ends that particular uncertainty (Fallowfield, 1991). Ramirez, Craig and Watson (1989) found that very threatening life events and difficulties were significantly associated with the first recurrence of breast cancer. Such results may suggest a prognostic association; however, Barraclough *et al.* (1992), studying over 200 patients, found no such association.

SEXUAL DIFFICULTIES

Sexual problems are common following breast cancer. There is often a loss of sexual interest and activity following mastectomy (Maguire *et al.*, 1978; Morris, Green and White, 1977) or after mastectomy or breast conservation treatment (Fallowfield, Baum and Maguire, 1986; Fallowfield, 1990), and these problems occur in at least 25% of patients. Sexual problems are also reported after chemotherapy, radiotherapy and hormone therapy.

ISOLATION AND THE NEED FOR SUPPORT

People who have cancer often experience a feeling of isolation; following her diagnosis, one patient wrote poignantly:

I felt immediately that I had entered a special place. This was the land of the sick people. The most disconcerting thing was not that I found the place so terrifying but that I found it so ordinary. I didn't feel different – what changed was other people's perception of me ... everyone regarded me as someone who has been altered irrevocably.

(Trillin, 1981)

At such times support may be vital.

EFFECTS ON PARTNERS, FAMILY AND FRIENDS

The impact breast cancer has on the patient's partner, family, friends, colleagues and even acquaintances can be severe and far-reaching. It can jeopardize what were previously open and trusting relationships because it is not an easy subject for discussion. Peters-Golden (1982) found that more than 50% of patients in her study felt that people avoided them, and 70% felt that their feelings of isolation were made more intense because of a lack of understanding by family and friends; 61% of healthy individuals felt they would try to avoid contact with a friend who had cancer.

Findings vary about the impact of breast cancer on those close to the patient. Cassileth, Luske and Strousse (1985) reported that if a patient was depressed or anxious there was a high probability their next of kin would be so as well. However, in a study of married couples, Hughes (1987) found that most people felt their relationship was the same or even enhanced following diagnosis and treatment for breast cancer. Only 11% of couples reported problems. However, Pistrong and Bartel (1992) reported that women felt less understood by partners than by friends and relatives.

Northouse (1990), analysing the effect of mastectomy on couples, found that while mood levels and role functioning improved over time, distress was still apparent 18 months later. There was a direct relationship between the couple's perceived lack of support and their distress levels.

Lewis, Ellison and Woods (1985) found that a mother's breast cancer was often stressful for her children, but Wellisch (1991) found that the daughters of women with breast cancer were not significantly more likely to have psychological problems than a control group. The effect of a mother's breast cancer on children's coping strategies was analysed by Issel, Erseck and Lewis (1990). They suggested that if clinicians understood these strategies they would be better able to facilitate the family's attempts to help.

For those who do allow themselves to become involved, it is difficult to avoid wanting to offer reassurances that may be false given the uncertain outcome of the disease. It is even more difficult to allow doubts about survival or coping to surface. Such doubts can trigger deep fears, not only in the patient and those close to her but also in those who are professionally involved in her care.

INFORMATION AND INFORMED CONSENT

There are numerous reports showing how dissatisfied patients are with the lack of adequate information about their disease, treatments and outcome (National Audit Commission, 1993). In one study (Anderson, 1988), patients undergoing mastectomy were interviewed; the great majority of them would have liked more information and guidance. Apart from the ethical, moral and legal reasons for providing patients with information (and yet not imposing it on those who do not want it), Fallowfield *et al.* (1990) showed that patients who perceived they had been well informed experienced less anxiety and depression, measured a year after diagnosis, than those who felt they had been inadequately informed. Cotton *et al.*, (1991) showed that patients who received information and support from a breast care nurse felt able to make decisions when offered a choice of treatment.

As well as receiving information from health care professionals in a medical setting, patients may also benefit from knowing about the various organizations that operate telephone helplines and distribute information, such as Breast Cancer Care (BCC, formerly the Breast Care and Mastectomy Association), British Association for Cancer United Patients (BACUP) and Cancerlink. BCC also operates a nationwide volunteer network, which can put a patient in touch with someone who has had the same experience and can act as a positive role model (Appendix A lists some useful addresses concerning information and support agencies).

The health care system in the USA operates differently, which may account for the fact that 75% of women in a recent study (Cawley, Kostic and Cappello, 1990), were satisifed with the information they received about lumpectomy for breast cancer. Significantly though, most of the satisfied women were in their 50s, whereas women in their 60s and 70s were less satisifed. Cawley, Kostic and Cappello suggested that older patients may be considered less capable of participating in major health care decisions and that a paternalistic approach is used more often in women in this age group.

The growth of the women's movement in the USA (and possibly to a lesser extent in the UK) has contributed to the lobby for government pressure to improve both research into the biology of breast cancer and the quality of the practical management of this disease.

The role of the nurse as the patient's advocate becomes particularly crucial when it comes to the matter of informed consent. Unless patients have adequate information they cannot give informed consent (or informed refusal) to treatment. This is particularly important in the current situation when there are many possible treatment options available but little consensus among health care professionals about which one to choose.

As a result of much lobbying by the public and organizations representing patients' interests (including the Breast Care Society at the Royal College of Nursing (RCN)), in 1990 the Department of Health issued guidelines

(DoH, 1990) that attempted to clarify the process of patient consent to treatment. The guidelines pay particular attention to consent for breast surgery: the patient is now required to sign to the effect that she completely understands the treatment that will follow. Importantly, the guidelines give patients the opportunity to state the nature of additional surgery that they do not want (such as not wishing a biopsy/frozen section to proceed to a mastectomy in the course of one operation). It is also suggested that patients may have a nurse or friend present when procedures are being explained.

Faulder (1985) defines valid informed consent as 'adequate disclosure from the informant met by adequate understanding from the person receiving the information, thus enabling the latter freely to give or refuse her consent'. Raphael (1988) brought to the public's attention the ethical difficulties that could arise when women were subjected to medical clinical trials, randomly being assigned to receive different treatments without their knowledge. Such dilemmas can also affect staff, whose loyalties are split between being accountable to the patient and yet being a member of a multidisciplinary team that may not be giving out adequate information (Feinmann, 1989).

Trying to manage the issues raised by informed consent is a complex, sensitive and emotive task. The role of the nurse in assisting the process of informed consent and acting as patient advocate was outlined by Tait (1989). Such a role has received support both from the United Kingdom Central Council (UKCC) advisory document *Exercising Accountability*, and the more detailed guidelines relating to the UKCC Code of Conduct (Burnard and Chapman, 1988).

Because of the many difficulties surrounding this area, the RCN Breast Care Nursing Society has produced a position statement to help those involved in care to clarify their roles. It includes the following points.

1. Patients cannot make decisions without relevant knowledge and opportunity for discussion being available. These are prerequisites for informed consent.
2. The nurse is required to act always in such a way as to promote and safeguard the wellbeing and interests of the patient/client. In breast care nursing this means the following:
   (a) As there is little consensus about the optimum treatments for breast cancer, it is vital that where relevant, options are discussed with the patient.
   (b) It is the nurse's responsibility to assess the patient's need for information and discussion and where it is required to ensure that these needs are met.
3. Once decisions are made, the nurse must act as the patient's advocate and defend her informed choice over whether to have treatment; opt for

one form of therapy over another; accept the medically recommended treatment; refuse treatment altogether.

4. If surgery is the treatment of choice, consent must again be informed. This requires investigative procedures to be followed by discussion before proceeding to surgery.

5. For other treatment modalities, it is the nurse's responsibility to ensure that the patient is aware of potential and certain side effects, and whether these are likely to be temporary or permanent.

6. Where clinical trials are in progress, it is the nurse's responsibility to assess the patient's understanding of her involvement and to make further information available as necessary.

It is important to remember, though, that some patients do not wish for information at all, and that those who do vary greatly in the amount they are prepared to take on board at a given time. Ley (1979) showed that patients seeing a doctor could only recall approximately 60% of the information given to them only 80 minutes after their consultation. However, Hogbin and Fallowfield (1989) showed that patients found a tape-recording of their 'bad news' consultation (at the time of diagnosis) to be extremely helpful. The presence of a relative or friend at the consultation, to aid recollection and provide support, can also be helpful.

MOOD DISTURBANCE

It is clear that between one-quarter and one-third of patients fail to adapt well to their diagnosis or treatment; because the incidence of breast cancer is so high, this proportion numbers a great many women (Graydon, 1982). Several studies have shown that approximately a quarter of women with breast cancer have significant psychological problems that usually benefit from detection and subsequent help, regardless of whether they have had a mastectomy or a partial removal of their breast plus radiotherapy (Dean, 1987; Fallowfield, Baum and Maguire, 1986; Fallowfield *et al.*, 1990; Maguire, 1994; Maguire *et al.*, 1978; Morris, Greer and White, 1977). The most common disorders are depressive illness and anxiety states, the two commonly coexisting. Sexual difficulties also frequently occur.

Anxiety states

An anxiety state or a depressive illness is different to the kind of mood disturbance that is a normal response to upsetting events. It is completely understandable that the traumatic experience of a diagnosis of breast cancer followed by treatment could result in much suffering; but such a view could lead health care professionals into believing that because it is understandable nothing needs to be done about it. It is therefore especially important to be clear about whether the mood changes a patient undergoes represent understandable unhappiness, such as a depressive or anxious reaction, or a significant response that merits treatment, such as a depressive illness or an anxiety state.

Diagnosing an anxiety state or a depressive illness can be difficult, depending on the adequate identification of particular signs and symptoms and their duration and frequency, as well as considering the patient's feelings. Usually such a state respresents a significant change from a patient's normal mood variations and it is often difficult to distract her from it, so there is often a lack of hope that the situation could change for the better. It is worth noting that few patients have trouble in distinguishing their normal from their abnormal mood, if asked. It is also worth noting that clinical depression and anxiety states require professional, specialized help.

Depressive illness

Hughes (1986) has outlined the following useful guidelines about depression.

- Both psychological and physical factors can be the precipitating cause of depressive illness and breast cancer patients may suffer multiple stresses because of the nature of its diagnosis and treatments.
- If patients do not have stable close relationships, adequate money, housing, or satisfying work, they are at increased risk.
- Although any personality type is vulnerable, those who have inflexible standards, are unduly dependent on others and are prone to mood swings are more likely to have depressive illness.

Watson (1991) also describes the vulnerability factors that may predict psychological morbidity. They are:

- Psychiatric history.
- Lack of support from family and friends.
- Pre-existing marital problems.
- Cancers and cancer treatments associated with visible deformity.
- Inability to accept the physical changes associated with the disease or its treatment.
- A younger age range.
- Tendency to suppress or contain negative feelings.
- Low expectation of efficacy of treatment.
- Lack of involvement in satisfying activities or occupation.
- More physical symptoms reported when cancer is diagnosed, regardless of the actual stage of the illness.
- An adverse experience of cancer in the family.
- Treatment by aggressive cytotoxic drugs.
- Additional concurrent stress.

It is important to distinguish between the physical symptoms caused by the depression and those caused by the disease process or treatments. Severe depressive episodes may result from changes in hormone and electrolyte metabolism, and are also a common symptom of organic brain disease, e.g. cerebral metastases. For this reason the mental symptoms of depressive illness may be more valuable in diagnosis than the physical ones.

The following is a checklist.

Mental symptoms

- A persistent lowering of mood for most of the time and for a duration of at least four weeks. It may show a diurnal variation, usually being worst in the morning and improving as the day goes on.
- This lowering of mood cannot be dispelled or diverted.
- A general lessening of interest and enjoyment in social or other activities.
- Sometimes crying takes place at the slightest provocation; sometimes patients want to cry, but feel frozen and unable to do so.
- A loss of interest in anything, poor concentration and an inability to enjoy pleasurable activities.
- Low self-esteem, feelings of worthlessness and a resulting lack of confidence.
- An exaggerated sense of guilt.
- Pessimism and hopelessness about the future, also suicidal thoughts.
- Anxiety and irritability.

Physical symptoms

- Sleep disturbance. Early waking is characteristic but there may also be difficulty getting off to sleep.
- Loss of appetite and loss of weight.
- Loss of energy and constant tiredness.
- Headaches or pains in other parts of the body.

It is thought that for a diagnosis of depressive illness at least four of the mental symptoms should be present and pervasive for a period of about four weeks, or, if these are not so apparent, if there are strongly suicidal thoughts.

Identifying anxiety states

It is natural for women with breast cancer and those who are involved with them to worry about it. However, unless the patient is in a state of acute anxiety and unable to function, an anxiety state can still be said to exist when such worries persist over time, for a period of at least four weeks, and are accompanied by at least four of the following (Wing, Cooper and Sartorious, 1974):

Mental symptoms

- Impaired concentration.
- Irritability and a feeling of being 'on edge'.

Physical symptoms

- Fatigueability.
- Sleep disturbance, such as difficulty getting off to sleep and/or waking throughout the night.
- Palpitations.
- Sweating.
- Frequency of micturition.
- Sudden panic attacks.
- Headaches or other tension pains.

There are other methods of measuring mood, such as questionnaires. Fallowfield (1990) describes several of these measures and advocates using the Hospital Anxiety and Depression scale devised by Zigmond and Snaith (1983) and the Rotterdam Symptom checklist (De Haes *et al.*, 1990).

COPING STRATEGIES

Coping means 'action directed at the resolution or mitigation of a problematic situation', according to Ray and Baum (1985). Experiencing the challenges mentioned so far has been shown to exact a heavy toll on patients. Consequently, rehabilitation – coping, for instance, with resuming relationships, household chores and returning to work – can be difficult.

However, the evidence suggests that most patients do cope well with their disease and treatment. For some, such an experience can even enhance their quality of life, giving a deeper meaning to their existence and relationships and a new sense of purpose (Ireland, 1987). Those who cope by sharing their worries, and who have a constructive and trusting attitude to those involved in their care, may be likely to adapt best (Weisman and Worden, 1977).

Morris, Greer and White (1977) and Greer and Watson (1987) have identified differing coping styles including:

- fighting spirit
- helplessness/hopelessness
- fatalism
- anxious preoccupation
- avoidance.

Such strategies may be difficult to categorize clinically, however. Since they are not mutually exclusive many patients will experience many styles of coping and may frequently be ambivalent about how they 'really' feel. Making value judgements about the merits of differing coping styles should be avoided.

The use of avoidance tactics or denial as a coping strategy may be misunderstood, for although it may be undesirable in some situations, such as delay in seeking a diagnosis, in other instances it can be a valuable defence that helps patients to cope better (Hughes, 1987).

Silberfarb, Maurer and Crouthameal (1980) regard 'adaptation' as a more suitable concept than 'coping' with regard to cancer. Adaptation focuses on the process of adjustment to what is often a chronic disease; thus adaptation is a way of managing a chronic state of uncertainty, rather than reacting to acute or dramatic events.

THE NEED FOR CRISIS INTERVENTION

However gradual adaptation may be, much of the management of patients is, in reality, focused around a crisis intervention strategy, the particular crisis being when the most acute stress is experienced.

According to Gorzynski (1982), the likely crisis times are:

- at the time of diagnosis or recurrence;
- following loss of a body part or function;
- when repeated side-effects or complications appear;
- when effective treatments have been exhausted;
- when social support fails.

A crisis is a situation that demands a response, 'It is not for subtle observation or contemplation' (Kennedy, 1989). The characteristics common to a person in crisis are:

- emotional shock;
- a need to change one's behaviour;
- a need for immediate action or intervention;
- the confrontation of a totally new phenomenon;
- the loss of the ability to think rationally or to integrate new information;
- a breakdown in the person's system of values;
- a feeling of having reached a 'dead end' with no sense of how to proceed;
- unpredictability – both for the person who experiences the crisis and those who observe the situation (Kfir, 1989).

It can be seen that all of these characteristics may be applicable to someone who is newly diagnosed with breast cancer.

REASONS WHY MANY PATIENTS' PROBLEMS ARE NOT IDENTIFIED OR MANAGED

Patients' reasons

Patients can apply harsh rules to themselves. They may be ashamed at being unable to cope emotionally and feel they should not be bothering staff who are busy and often overworked. They may feel their suffering is understandable and that nothing can be done about it anyway. Also, since staff do not routinely ask them about psychosocial problems, tending to focus on physical difficulties, patients may think that such concerns are not legitimate.

Staff reasons

There are several reasons why staff may not identify patients' problems. Firstly, there is evidence of a deficit in communication skills in nursing in general (Faulkner, 1980; Macleod Clarke, 1982) and in cancer nursing in particular (Bond, 1982; Wikinson, 1991). There is also considerable evidence of problems with other health care professionals, including doctors (Maguire and Faulkner, 1988).

These studies showed that those involved in care often avoided answering difficult questions, failed to pick up 'cues' signalling distress and used blocking tactics to control conversations with patients. The distancing tactics that were commonly used included the following.

Selective attention to cues

Nurse: How have you been?
Patient: Well, they say my scar is healing, but I'm worried.
Nurse: It's great that your scar is better. Now let's see when we need to organize your first prosthesis fitting, and if you like I'll tell you about the different kinds we stock.

The clue that was concerned with feelings and might have been of great significance – 'but I'm worried' – was ignored because the nurse found it safer to comment on the physical symptom of the scar and on the offer of practical help. In that way she could be seen to be 'doing something'.

Switching of topics

Patient: I'm wondering why I have lost weight lately.
Nurse: Are you going to sit out of bed now?

This neglect of the patient's concerns could have been avoided if the nurse had reflected back what the patient had said and then clarified what the concern was:

Nurse: You sounded a bit concerned about your weight, can you tell me a bit more about that?

'Inappropriate' reassurance

Premature reassurance before identifying what the patient's concerns are:

Patient: I feel scared now I'm actually in here.

Nurse: There's no need to, we'll take good care of you, Mr Smith is an excellent surgeon and very understanding.

The nurse could have stayed 'tuned in' to the patient's feelings about being scared:

Nurse: You say that you're scared; can you perhaps tell me what it is that you are so scared about?

False reassurance:

Nurse: We'll soon have you forgetting you ever had this operation.

This nurse made a promise that she or he could not be sure of keeping.

Closed questions

Closed questions, when the nurse is suggesting the answer she wants to hear, or 'setting the agenda':

Nurse: You don't seem to be feeling so bad today, do you?

Although it might be hoped that such tactics were a thing of the past, in her study of nurses interviewing cancer patients, Wilkinson (1991) showed that such problems still exist.

Sometimes problems occur because of the 'inappropriate' nature of the subject matter of conversations with patients. Although there is an increasing tendency in many areas of life for public comments on personal and intimate matters, Faulkner (1986) has postulated that the content of professional interaction is different from most social exchange.

Many of the subjects raised would, in another context, be socially taboo. These include seuxality, death and dying, fear provoking diagnosis and prognosis, body image and bodily functions.

These are precisely the subjects that are likely to be of concern to the patient at different stages in the process of her breast cancer. If the patient is to feel it is legitimate to discuss them, the nurse must 'give permission', tuning in to any cues the patient has already offered, or raising such issues herself by appropriate, sensitive questioning.

Wilkinson also showed that good communication was not just a matter of having the necessary communication skills; knowledge about cancer and its treatment (e.g. having undertaken a relevant advanced English National Board (ENB) course) also contributed to an improved level of practice. Additionally the environment in which care took place (e.g. the management style and atmosphere of openness and trust created by the ward sister or other influential figure in the hierarchy) also mattered.

These findings have been borne out by Smith (1992), who found that the emotional style of the ward sister greatly affected the nurses' ability to care for the psychological needs of patients, and that the 'emotional labour' that was an integral part of the nurses' role often had scant attention or support from nurse educators or clinical managers.

Some studies indicate that in addition to the lack of specialist knowledge, good communication skills and an enabling environment, many health care staff tend to protect themselves from the personal pain they might experience if they come too close to the suffering of individual patients. In a classic study of hospital life, Menzies (1988) showed how the organization of nursing work was compartmentalized into tasks, thus stopping nurses from providing continuity of care or having too close a relationship with patients. Menzies felt that this organization was deliberate, intended not to help patients but to protect nurses from anxiety.

Doctors and nurses may not realize that they block communication. Writing about her experiences as a breast care nurse, Tait (1990) analysed her own interview with a patient and realized how she had blocked difficult questions. She wrote: 'These were attempts to cope with the moment – not coming too close to matters of life and death, which frightened me as much as the patients'. Once the patient has been encouraged to unleash powerful emotions, it can be difficult for staff to know how best to proceed in the interests of either the patient or themselves.

COMMUNICATION

There are varying views about what particular activities terms such as communication, assessment and counselling comprise. Macleod Clarke, Hopper and Jesson (1991) have defined the differences between them by describing them as a hierarchy of activities in the shape of a pyramid. At the broad base lies communication skills, which include assessment, giving information and advice, as well as the opportunity for discussion and expression of feelings.

Assessment

The continuing assessment of a patients' ability to cope or adapt is vital for the patient and her family, yet although there is an increasing awareness of this need, it is not yet practised adequately by many of those involved in care (Maguire, 1985; Tait, 1994). An assessment is needed to identify patients' problems as they perceive them.

The crucial area of assessment – that of the patient's physical, psychological and social problems and needs – requires not only good communication skills, but also knowledge of the particular topics that previous research has shown to be important in commonly-experienced problems.

The structure, content and methods of assessment of patients who have had mastectomy have been described by Tait *et al* (1982). However, the basic format is relevant to all patients with breast cancer whatever their surgical or other treatment. The order in which topics are raised can vary, so that patients can volunteer particular areas of concern and thus prioritize their own needs. However, the fact that there is the opportunity for the nurse to make sensitive enquiries about topics the patient may not have mentioned, gives the patient 'permission' to talk about them if she wishes to.

The topics that should be covered at appropriate stages of the patient's disease process include:

- The patient's view of her disease and treatment.
- Previous experience of cancer (especially breast cancer) in others.
- Other recent stressful events, apart from breast cancer.
- The impact of her disease and treatment on:
  relationships with significant people in her life including her partner and family;
  sexuality;
  body image;
  spiritual philosophy;
  mood state, including anxiety and depression;
  work, including relationships with colleagues;
  finances;
  social life, including friendships, hobbies and interests;
  housework, including chores and shopping.
- Coping strategies.

Patients' perceptions of these matters may vary both individually and culturally. If the nurse is introducing a potentially sensitive topic, such as how a patient may be feeling about her relationship with her partner, it is important to start with a general open question asked in a tentative way, so that the patient can easily stop the conversation if she finds it intrusive. For example, a general question might be:

You were mentioning your partner, do you mind if I ask you, how do you feel you are getting on at the moment?

If the patient is happy to talk about him or her, it may then be appropriate to focus on whether the disease or treatment appears to be causing any significant change in the relationship.

Using good assessment techniques – asking relevant questions, picking up cues, focusing on the patient's expressed concerns and encouraging the expression of feelings – enables the nurse to legitimize the discussion of psychosocial problems. By 'getting close' she or he can also clearly demonstrate how much she or he cares.

Assessment of functional status after diagnosis of breast cancer is advocated by Tulman and Fawcett (1990) in relation to a woman's role as wife, mother, home-maker, community member and worker. The need for adequate assessment of psychosexual needs following minimal surgery, such as lumpectomy, as well as after mastectomy, is stressed by Rutherford (1988).

COUNSELLING

Counselling, as defined by the British Association of Counselling (BAC), is an interaction in which one person offers another time, attention and respect with the intention of helping that person to explore, discover and clarify ways of living more resourcefully and towards greater well-being (BAC, 1989).

It is worth noting that during counselling the patient has an active role in working through her problems for herself. To do this, she requires skilled support, but not necessarily advice. Consequently, once assessment of need has taken place it may be possible for the nurse, after further training and self-awareness of his or her own attitudes and beliefs, to use counselling skills to facilitate the patient in a deeper exploration of the issues arising from the illness. However, use of such skills does not, in itself, produce a 'counsellor'. In the view of Macleod Clarke, Hopper and Jesson (1991), to become a qualified counsellor a nurse must have undertaken a recognized training programme as well as needing to receive supervision of her client caseload from another experienced counsellor or psychotherapist.

Counselling at this level usually requires patient and nurse to negotiate a contract and to have a fixed number of sessions. However, the nurse's role generally is to help with problems related to the disease process or its treatments, not to change a patient's attitudes and behaviour concerning other matters.

WHO WANTS HELP?

Although it is generally accepted that everyone may benefit from good communication, it is important to realize that some people prefer not to enter into long or deep discussions; they may simply not want to, or they may not be used to articulating their concerns. Furthermore, research has already demonstrated that denial may at times be a useful coping mechanism.

It is particularly important that assumptions are not made about a general need for counselling as this could result in conflict with a patient's right to privacy and self-determination. In addition to those who want (and have a right) to manage their problems themselves, patients with certain kinds of mental or physical illness, such as brain damage, strong defence mechanisms or severe depression, cannot be effectively counselled.

THE RESEARCH BASE FOR PSYCHOSOCIAL CARE

Research evidence shows that the strategies for breast care nursing identified so far in this chapter can significantly benefit patients. In one study (Maguire *et al.*, 1983), a control group of patients undergoing mastectomy had routine care alone. The experimental group of patients had access to a specialist nurse, trained to assess them for evidence of depressive illness, anxiety states and sexual problems.

Although the presence of the nurse did not actually prevent patients experiencing anxiety, depression and sexual problems, there were some positive results. Those who had access to the nurse achieved a better social adjustment, returned to work sooner and were more satisfied with their breast prosthesis. Another positive result was that the nurse recognized 76% of the women in her group who had developed significant psychological problems. In the majority of cases they were referred for psychological therapy. In the control group of patients who had routine care alone, psychological problems were recognized or referred on in only 15% of those who developed them. As a result of this difference in care the experimental group had three times less anxiety and depression than the control group at the end of the year following surgery (Maguire *et al.*, 1980a).

At the end of this study the researchers concluded that it may have been naive to have supposed that having a nurse monitoring patients' progress, giving them information, practical advice and emotional support, plus referring some patients to other specialist resource people would have been adequate to prevent patients from having significant psychological problems. However, implicit in any such project is the hope that this might be the outcome.

Some other difficulties were encountered in this study. The specialist nurse had initiated contact at regular intervals during the year following surgery. Some patients were made more anxious by the continuing nursing assessments, perhaps because they wanted to forget their breast cancer and treatments. It was realized that some patients would prefer to try and cope without help, and that targeting help to those who wanted it was more appropriate so long as strategies could be identified to indicate those who might require it. Some patients became dependent on the nurse for matters unrelated to breast cancer.

Following this study, the cost-benefits of employing the specialist nurse were studied by a team including researchers from a health services management unit (Maguire *et al.*, 1982). The findings of this study showed that patients in both the control and the experimental group suffered considerable financial losses, but that these were offset for patients in the experimental group by their earlier return to work. The researchers concluded that the specialist nurse scheme was necessary and effective and could be implemented at little extra cost.

All these considerations led to another research study being funded by the then Department of Health and Social Security (now the Department of Health). This randomized controlled clinical trial was carried out to see what the psychological outcome was for patients in three differing groups (Wilkinson, Maguire and Tait, 1988). The study compared the intervention of specialist nurses with that of non-specialist (i.e. ward and community) nurses, with patients who had breast cancer. It also compared the patient outcome of specialist nurses using unlimited intervention (i.e. regular follow-up) with only limited intervention (i.e. one home visit, then leaving the onus on the patient to contact the nurse).

As in the first study, counselling failed to prevent psychiatric morbidity, but the results of this more complex study were otherwise not so clear cut. They were useful in that they showed that limited intervention by specialist nurses was as effective in identifying and managing (often by referral) psychological morbidity as was continual follow-up. Even so, patients in the limited intervention group were not significantly better in the areas of physical or social recovery. One useful finding was that, so long as the nurse could convey her interest and motivation to help the patient, and was readily accessible and available, most patients were well able to make contact and seek help.

The results also showed that the ward nurses were better able to identify psychological problems than the community nurses and that specialist nurses were significantly more likely to recognize and refer psychological problems than either the ward or community groups. However, some of the results in this study showed no significant differences among the three main groups because even within one group (i.e. the specialist nurse's) there was a considerable variation in performance.

Partly as a result of this study it has been argued that if the ability to monitor psychological problems can be taken on by non-specialist nurses, specalist nurses may then be released to motivate, educate and support the non-specialist nurses and other health care professionals, so becoming a significant resource to staff as well as direct care-givers to patients.

The explanations offered for the results were that the ward nurses, who performed better than the community nurses, might have done so because they were part of a cohesive group and also their managers happened to value and support this work. Much of community work takes place on an individual basis and managers may not necessarily see the value, given the amount of other work there is to do, of psychological monitoring of breast cancer patients (Faulkner and Maguire, 1984; Faulkner and Maguire, 1990).

Another evaluation of a specialist nurse service was undertaken by Watson and co-workers in 1988. Following mastectomy, patients were randomized to receive routine care alone or routine care plus counselling by a specialist nurse. Comparisons between the groups indicated that counselled patients were significantly less depressed three months post-operatively and reported more beliefs in personal control over health. At 12 months post-operatively there were no significant differences between the groups, although patients' adjustment throughout the year following surgery occurred more rapidly if they were counselled by the specialist nurse.

One aspect of this study was that the specialist nurse intervention started at the time of a patint receiving her diagnosis, earlier than in the previous studies quoted. The effect of this early intervention may have contributed to the significant difference between the two groups at the three-month post-diagnosis assessment. The positive results led the researchers to conclude that a nurse counselling service was of value in reducing the amount of distress experienced as a result of the diagnosis and treatment of breast cancer.

As a result of all these research findings, a simple framework for psychological care has developed based on the core skills of communication, assessment and counselling advocated by Maguire. Many breast care nurses use this basic framework and find it relevant to their practice (Tait, 1994). Some then develop their skills further and become qualified counsellors as well.

One of the most important aspects of nursing care, vital to all the studies quoted above, was the ability of the nurse to recognize her or his own limitations regarding the provision of specialized psychological therapy and her/his ability to identify and refer patients with particular needs (eg. significant anxiety and depression) to other specialists. However, if a nurse has not been able to identify psychological resource people, she or he may well feel there is no point in picking up a patient's problems, because nothing can be done about them anyway.

THE USE OF PARTICULAR THERAPIES

There have been varying results from studies evaluating particular forms of intervention by other health care professionals. One study (Spiegel *et al.*, 1989) analysed the survival outcome of women with metastatic breast cancer, randomized to receive routine care alone or supportive group counselling and self-hypnosis. A significant survival advantage to the counselled group was shown.

Greer *et al.* (1992) reported a study that compared patients having routine care alone with a group having brief adjuvant psychological therapy using a problem focused and cognitive/behavioural treatment programme specifically designed for the needs of individual patients. Treated patients achieved significantly lower scores for anxiety, psychological symptoms and psychological distress four months following treatment. The long-term effects are not yet known, however.

Tarrier, Maguire and Vincey (1984) also found a marked improvement in patients' self-confidence and self-esteem when cognitive therapy, i.e. structured methods to change negative thinking and behaviour, were used. They found that a combination of antidepressant medication and cognitive therapy also alleviated depression. The management of depression is usefully discussed by Hughes (1986) who also advocates a counselling approach combined with antidepressant drugs in many cases.

Bridges *et al.* (1988) showed that a structured programme of relaxation and visualization for an experimental group of patients having radiotherapy for primary breast cancer was significantly more effective in alleviating psychological distress than the unstructured 'chat' given to patients in the control group.

VOLUNTEERS AND SELF-HELP GROUPS

For some patients, meeting someone who has had similar experiences and problems and who has overcome them can be of great benefit, and many patients have been helped in this way. However, if volunteers are to be effective they should be chosen carefully so that they do not damage themselves or others (Mantell, 1983).

Volunteers require some degree of self-awareness so that they do not impose their own experiences on others, but rather develop the ability to 'tune in' to their client's problems. In order to feel and be more secure they should work within accepted guidelines and boundaries. Volunteers will consequently require some training, but not so much that they become 'mini-professionals' and lose what they uniquely have to offer as a positive role model. Training and support can safeguard the volunteer as well as her client. Breast Cancer Care (Breast Care and Mastectomy Association, 1991) is developing such work.

Similarly, support and self-help groups can be very beneficial, but the same kind of rules apply. A lack of proper training, leadership, structure and support may damage those who offer help as well as those requiring it. However, the fact that so many groups exist and flourish is a testimony to the need for their existence (Trojan, 1989). Help in setting up and managing groups can be obtained from Cancerlink (address details in Appendix A).

THE SEARCH FOR MEANING

Part of the supportive counselling that may be offered to patients who want it concerns their search for meaning, their attempt to try to make sense of their diagnosis, illness and, perhaps, impending death. O'Connor (1990) has outlined major themes in this process, including trying to understand the personal significance of the diagnosis (the 'why me?' analysis), a review of life, a change in outlook towards self and others, and living with cancer and hope.

George (1990), in discussing the counselling work of specialist breast care nurses, suggests that for some patients an existential philosophy may provide a map of the differing dimensions in life through which people travel, such as the physical/biological, the public/social, the private feelings/aspirations and the spiritual beliefs/values. By doing this work, a patient can be taught how to recognize and understand her emotional life, so gaining a sense of mastery over it. Such mastery may enable patients to understand that disease process must be integrated into the general life process, as opposed to actually being the life process. However, for such therapy to be effective George suggests that the counsellor must have some clarity and self-awareness about her own professional and personal assumptions on life and living before being able to help others make sense of their lives.

> Clients are entitled to a counsellor who has grappled with the essential issues and questions that life raises.

But how much training is a nurse likely to have had in such an important area?

A crucial component of most accredited counselling courses is experiential and theoretical training in self-awareness. In a survey by Roberts and Fallowfield (1990), many nurses who specialized in cancer 'counselling' did not have formal qualifications in this subject and few had supervision by psychologically-qualified health care professionals. The reasons for these findings and details about intended counselling training were not explored, however. Many specialist breast care nurses have had or intend to have some training in counselling skills and some are actively seeking professional supervision of their work by effective, psychologically trained professionals (Tait 1994). They also seek professionals to whom patients may be referred for psychological therapy, although sometimes supervision and referral cannot take place because of a shortage of adequate resources.

The importance of adequate support for both the patient and the nurse is well recognized. Yasco (1983), for instance, found that lack of psychological support was a significant predictor of burn-out in nursing. Even so the important question of who may give it remains. It is important for the nurse to have insight into her own situation (Vachon and Lyall, 1978) but also for nurse managers and other clinicians to understand and support this requirement.

It is likely that no one mechanism for support would meet a nurse's total needs. It must be understood that a patient's behaviour and attitudes do not just reside 'objectively' in the patient, but are in part constructed by those with whom patients interact. The way a nurse defines a patient's behaviour and reacts to it could well be the product of her own fears and anxieties, perhaps because of the emotive nature of breast cancer. If these concerns are allowed to surface and are accepted, and adequate support is given, the quality of the experience for both patient and nurse is likely to be improved.

REFERENCES

Anderson, J. (1988) Facing up to mastectomy. *Nursing Times,* **84**, 36–9.

Anderson, J. (1989) The nurse's role in cancer rehabilitation. Review of the literature. *Cancer Nursing,* **12**(2), 85–94.

BAC (1989) *British Association of Counselling Training Directory.* British Association of Counselling, Rugby.

Badwe, R., Gregory, W., Chaudary, M. *et al.* (1991) Timing of the menstrual cycle and survival of pre-menopausal women with operable breast cancer. *The Lancet,* 1261–4.

Bagenal, F., Easton, D., Harris, E. *et al.* (1990) Survival of patients with breast cancer attending Bristol Cancer Help Centre. *The Lancet,* 606–8.

Bard, M. and Sutherland, A. (1952) Psychologial impact of cancer and its treatment (iv) Adaptation to radical mastectomy. *Cancer,* **8**, 652–72.

Barraclough, J., Pinder, P., Cruddas, M. *et al.* (1992) Life events and breast cancer prognosis. *British Medical Journal,* **304**, 1078–81.

Beaver, K., Luter, K., Leinster, S., Owens, R. (1994) Preferences for information and decision making in women newly diagnosed with breast cancer. *Report to the Research in Cancer Nursing Conference,* King's College, London.

Bloom, J. (1982) Social support, accommodation to stress and adjustment to breast cancer. *Social Science and Medicine,* **16**; 1329–38.

Bond, S. (1982) Communications in Cancer Nursing, in *Cancer Nursing* (ed. M. Cahoon), Churchill-Livingstone, London.

Breast Care and Mastectomy Association (1991) *Annual Report,* Breast Care and Mastectomy Association, London.

Bridges, L., Benson, L., Pietroni, P. and Priest, C. (1988) Relaxation and imagery in the treatment of breast cancer. *British Medical Journal,* **297**, 1169–72.

Brohn, P. (1987) *The Bristol Programme. An introduction to the holistic therapies practised by the Bristol cancer help centre,* Century, London.

Burnard, P. and Chapman, C. (1988) *Professional and Ethical Issues in Nursing. The Code of Professional Conduct,* John Wiley & Sons, Chichester.

Cancer Relief Macmillan Fund (1994) *Breast Cancer. How to help yourself.* C.R.M.F.

Cassileth, B., Lusk, E. and Strousse, T. (1985) A psychological analysis of cancer patients and their next of kin. *Cancer,* **55**, 72–6.

Cawley, M., Kostic, J. and Cappello, C. (1990) Information and psychosocial needs of women choosing conservative surgery/primary radiation for early stage breast cancer. *Cancer Nursing,* **13**, February, 90–4.

Clyne, R. (1989) *Cancer – Your Life, Your Choice,* Thorsons, Wellingborough.

Consensus Development Conference; Treatment of Primary Breast Cancer (1986) *British Medical Journal,* **293**, 946–7.

Cotton, T., Locker, A., Jackson, L. *et al.* (1991) A prospective study of patient choice in treatment for primary breast cancer. *European Journal of Surgical Oncology,* **17**, 115–17.

Dean, C. (1987) Psychiatric morbidity following mastectomy. *Journal of Psychosomatic Research,* **31**, 385–92.

Degner, L. and Sloan, J. (1992) Decision making during serious illness: what role do patients really want to play? *Journal of Clinical Epidemiology,* **45**(9), 941–50.

Denton, S. and Baum, M. (1982) Can we predict which women will fail to cope with mastectomy? *Clinical Oncology*, **8**, 375–9.

De Haes, J., Knippenberg, F., Neift, J. (1990) Measuring psychological and physical distress in cancer patients: structure and application of the Rotterdam Sympton Check test. *British Journal of Cancer*, **62**, 1034–8.

Department of Health (1990) A guide to consent for examination or treatment, HMSO, London.

Department of Health (1994) Consultative Document. *A Policy Framework for Commissioning Cancer Services*, H.M.S.O.

Fallowfield, L. (1990) *The Quality of Life. The missing measurement in health care*, Human horizons series, Souvenir Press, London.

Fallowfield, L. (1991) *Breast Cancer*, Routledge, London.

Fallowfield, L., Baum, M. and Maguire, G.P. (1986) Effects of breast conservation on psychological morbidity associated with diagnosis and treatment of early breast cancer. *British Medical Journal*, **293**, 1331–4.

Fallowfield, L., Hall, A., Maguire, G.P. and Baum, M. (1990) Psychological outcomes of different treatment policies in women with early breast cancer outside a clinical trial. *British Medical Journal*, **301**, 575–80.

Faulder, C. (1985) *Whose body is it? The Troubling Issue of Informed Consent*, Virago, London.

Faulkner, A. (1980) The student nurse's role in giving information to patients. University of Aberdeen M. Litt. Thesis.

Faulkner, A. (1986) Talking to patients. Human Interest. *Nursing Times*, **82**(33), 33–5.

Faulkner, A. and Maguire, G.P. (1984) Teaching assessment skills, in *Recent Advances in Nursing 7. Communication* (ed. A. Faulkner) Churchill Livingstone, Edinburgh.

Faulkner, A. and Maguire, G.P. (1990) Assessing cancer patients in the community, in *Oncology* (ed. A. Faulkner), Scutari press, London.

Feinman, J. (1989) Consent on Trial. *Nursing Times*. **84**(44), 20.

Fentiman, I. and Mansel, R. (1991) The axilla: not a no-go zone. *The Lancet*, **337**, 221–3.

George, D. (1990) An existential perspective on the anxiety inherent in the role of the clinical nurse specialist in breast cancer. Department of Psychology, Antioch University, London, MA thesis.

Gorzynski, J. (1982) Depression in cancer patients: prevalence, diagnosis and psychotropic drug management. *Current Concepts in Psychosocial Oncology*, Memorial Sloan-Kettering Cancer Centre, New York.

Graydon, J. (1982) Aspects of Breast Cancer, in *Cancer Nursing* (ed. M.C. Cahoon), Churchill-Livingstone, Edinburgh.

Greer, S. (1990) Fighting spirit as a prognostic variable in cancer. *British Journal of Hospital Medicine* (Conference supplement: Cancer and the mind), 22–3.

Greer, S., Moorey, S., Baruch, J. *et al.* (1992) Adjuvant psychological therapy for patients with cancer: a prospective randomised trial. *British Medical Journal*, **304**, 675–80.

Greer, S. and Watson, M. (1987) Mental adjustment to cancer, its measurement and prognostic importance. *Cancer Surveys*, **6**, 439–53.

Halls, A., Fallowfield, L., Baum, M., Maguire, P., A'Hern, R. (1994) Psychological impact on recurrent breast cancer. *Report of the British Psychosocial Oncology Group Conference.* December.

Hogbin, B. and Fallowfield, L. (1989) Getting it taped: the 'bad news' consultation with cancer patients. *British Journal of Hospital Medicine*, **41**, 330–3.

Hopwood, P. (1984) Measurement of psychological morbidity in cancer, in *Psychosocial issues in malignant disease* (eds M. Watson and S. Greer), Pergamon Press, Oxford.

House of Commons (1991) A breast care nurse in every health district, health board and screening assessment centre. *Early day motion*.

Hughes, J. (1986) Depression in cancer patients, in *Coping with Cancer Stress* (ed. B. Stoll), Martinus Nijhoff, Chichester.

Hughes, J. (1987) *Cancer and emotion*, John Wiley & Sons, Chichester.

Hughson, A., Cooper, A., McArdle, C. and Smith, D. (1987) Psychological impact of adjuvant chemotherapy in the first two years after mastectomy. *British Medical Journal*, **293**, 1265–71.

Ireland, J. (1987) *Life wish*, Century, London.

Issel, M., Erseck, M. and Lewis, F. (1990) How children cope with mother's breast cancer. *Oncology Nursing Forum*. 17(**3**), supplement, 5–12.

Kennedy, E. (1989) *Crisis Counselling*, Gill and Macmillan, Southampton.

Kfir, N. (1989) *Crisis Intervention Verbatim*, Hemisphere, London.

Knopf, A. (1974) *Cancer. Changes in opinion after seven years of public education in Lancaster*, Manchester Regional Committee Report.

Lewis, F., Ellison, E. and Woods, N. (1985) The impact of breast cancer on the family. *Seminars Oncology Nursing*, **3**, 206–13.

Ley, P. (1979) Memory and medicine information. *British Journal of Social and Clinical Psychology*, **8**, 245–55.

Lorde, A. (1980) *The Cancer Journals*, Sheba Feminist Publishers, London.

Lucas, D., Maguire, G.P. and Reason, J. (1987) *Predicting psychiatric morbidity in women with breast cancer*. Report of the North West Regional Health Authority, Manchester.

Macleod Clarke, J. (1982) Nurse–patient verbal interaction. University of London PhD thesis.

Macleod Clarke, J., Hopper, L. and Jesson, A. (1991) Progression to counselling. *Nursing Times*. **87**(8), 41–3.

Maguire, G.P. (1976) The Psychological and Social Sequelae of Mastectomy, in *Modern Perspectives in the Psychiatric Aspects of Surgery* (ed. J. Howells), Churchill-Livingstone, Edinburgh.

Maguire, G.P. (1985) Barriers to psychological care of the dying. *British Medical Journal*, **291**, 1711–13.

Maguire, P. (1994) Psychological Aspects in A.B.C. of Breast Diseases, *British Medical Journal*, **309**, 1649–52.

Maguire, G.P., Brooke, M., Tait, A. *et al.* (1983) The effect of counselling on physical disability and social recovery after mastectomy. *Clinical Oncology*, 9, 319–21.

Maguire, G.P. and Faulkner, A. (1988) How to do it. Improve the counselling skills of doctors and nurses in cancer care. *British Medical Journal*, **297**, 847–9.

Maguire, G.P., Lee, E., Bevingdon, D. *et al.* (1978) Psychiatric problems in the first year after mastectomy. *British Medical Journal*, **1**, 963–5.

Maguire, G.P., Pentol, A., Allen, D. *et al.* (1982) Cost of counselling women who undergo mastectomy. *British Medical Journal*, **284**, 1933–5.

Maguire, G.P., Tait, A., Brooke, M. *et al.* (1980a). The effects of counselling on the psychiatric morbidity associated with mastectomy. *British Medical Journal*, **281**, 1454–6.

Maguire, G.P., Tait, A., Brooke, M. *et al.* (1980b) Psychiatric morbidity and physical toxicity associated with adjuvant chemotherapy after mastectomy. *British Medical Journal*, ii, 1179–80.

Maguire, G.P. and Sellwood, R. (1982) A liaison psychiatry service for mastectomy patients in *A Handbook of Liaison Psychiatry* (eds F. Creed and J. Pfeffer), Pitman Medical, London.

Mantell, J. (1983) Cancer patients visitor programs. A case for accountabilty. *Journal of Psychosocial Oncology*, **1**, 45.

McCaffrey, D. (1991) Surviving Cancer. *Nursing Times*, **87**(32), 26–9.

Menzies, I. (1988) A case study of the functioning of social systems as a defence against anxiety. The report on a study of a nursing service of a general hospital, in *Containing Anxiety in Institutions* (ed. I. Menzies), Free Association Books, London.

Miller, M. and Nygren, B. (1978) Living with cancer coping behaviors. *Cancer Nursing*, **4**, 297–302.

Morris, J. and Royle, G. (1987) Offering patients a choice of surgery for early breast cancer. A reduction in anxiety and depression in patients and their husbands. *Social Science and Medicine*, **26**(6), 583–5.

Morris, T. (1983) Psychosocial Aspects of Breast Cancer; a Review. *European Journal of Clinical Oncology*, **19**(12), 1725–33.

Morris, T., Greer, S. and White, P. (1977) Psychological and social adjustment to mastectomy. *Cancer*, **40**, 2381–7.

National Audit Commission for Local Authorities and the National Health Servicein England and Wales (1993) '*What seems to be the matter?*' *Communication between hospitals and patients*, HMSO.

Northouse, L. (1990) A longitudinal study of the adjustment of patients and husbands to breast cancer. *The Oncology Nursing Forum*, **17**(3), supplement, 39–43.

O'Connor, (1990) Understanding the cancer patient's search for meaning. *Cancer Nursing*, **13**(3), 167–75.

Peck, A. and Boland, J. (1977) Emotional reactions to radiation treatment. *Cancer*, **40**, 180–4.

Penman, D., Bloom, J., Fotopouloss, S. *et al.* (1988) The impact of mastectomy on self concept and social function, a combined cross sectional and longitudinal study with comparison groups, in *Women and Cancer* (ed. S. Stellman), The Howarth Press, London.

Peters-Golden, H. (1982) Breast Cancer: varied perceptions of social support in the illness experience. *Social Science and Medicine*, **16**, 483–91.

Pistrong, N. and Barker, C. (1992) Disclosures of Concerns in Breast Cancer. *Psycho-oncology*, **1**(3), 183–92.

Plumb, M. and Holland, J. (1981) Comparative studies of psychological function in patients with advanced cancer. (ii) Interviewer rated current and past psychiatric symptoms. *Psychosomatic Medicine*, **43**, 243–54.

Prior, S. (1987) Personal View. *British Medical Journal*, **295**, 920.

Quint, J. (1964) Mastectomy – symbol of cure or warning sign? *General Practitioner*, March, 119–25.

Ramirez, A., Craig, T. and Watson, J. (1989) Stress and relapse of breast cancer. *British Medical Journal*, **298**, 291–3.

Raphael, A. (1988) How doctors' secret trials abused me. *The Observer*, 9 October, 12.

Ray, C. and Baum, M. (1985) *Psychological aspects of early breast cancer*, Springer-Verlag, New York.

RCN Standards (1994) *Breast Care Nursing Society Standards of Care*, Royal College of Nursing.

Roberts, R. and Fallowfield, L. (1990) Who supports the cancer counsellors? *Nursing Times* **86**(36), 32–4.

Rosser, J. (1981) The interpretation of women's experience; a critical appraisal of the literature on breast cancer. *Social Science and Medicine*, **15**, 257–65.

Rutherford, (1988) Assessing psychosexual needs of women experiencing lumpectomy. *Cancer Nursing*, **11**(4), 244–9.

Silberfarb, P., Maurer, H. and Crouthameal, C. (1980) Psychosocial aspects of neo-plastic disease. 1. Functional status of breast cancer patients during different treatment regimes. *American Journal of Psychiatry*, **1374**, 450–5.

Smith, P. (1992) *The Emotional Labour of Nursing. How nurses care*, Macmillan, London.

Sontag, S. (1979) *Illness as Metaphor*, Penguin Books, London.

Spiegel, D., Bloom, J., Kraemer, H. and Gottheil, E. (1989) The effect of psychosocial treatment on survival of patients with metastatic breast cancer. *The Lancet*, 886–91.

Tait, A. (1989) Informed consent. Nursing Practice. *Nursing Standard* (oncology supplement), **36**(3), 55.

Tait, A. (1990) The Mastectomy Experience, in *Feminist Praxis. Research theory and epistimology in feminist sociology* (ed. L. Stanley), Routledge, London.

Tait, A. (1994) *Breast Care Nursing*, Report to Cancer Relief Macmillan Fund.

Tait, A., Maguire, G., Brook, M. *et al.* (1982) Improving communication skills. Standardized assessments for mastectomy patients. *Nursing Times*, **78**(51), 2181–4.

Tarrier, N., Maguire, G.P. and Kincey, J. (1984) Treatment of psychological distress following mastectomy; an initial report. *Behavioural Research and Therapy*, **22**, 81.

Trillin, A. (1981) Of dragons and garden peas: a cancer patient talks to doctors. *New England Journal of Medicine*, **304**, 699–701.

Trojan, S. (1989) Benefits of Self Help Groups. *Social Science and Medicine*, **29**(2), 225–32.

Tulman, L. and Fawcett, J. (1990) A framework for studying functional status after diagnosis of breast cancer. *Cancer Nursing*, **13**(2), 95–9.

Vachon, M. and Lyall, W. (1978) Management of stress in health professionals working with advanced cancer patients. *Death Education*, **1**, 365–75.

Watson, M. (1991) Breast Cancer, in *Cancer Patient Care, Psychosocial Treatment Methods* (ed. M. Watson), British Psychological Society, Cambridge University Press, Cambridge.

Watson, M., Denton, S., Baum, M. and Greer, S. (1988) Counselling breast cancer patients – a specialist nurse service. *Counselling Psychology Quarterly*, **1**(1), 23–31.

Weisman, A. (1979) *Coping with cancer*, McGraw-Hill, New York.

Weisman, A., Worden, J. (1977) Coping and vulnerability in cancer patients. *Project Omega Report*, Department of Psychiatry, Harvard Medical School, Boston.

Welch-McCaffrey, D. (1985) Evolving patient education needs in cancer. *Oncology Nursing Forum*, **12**, 62–6.

Wellisch, D. (1991) *Psychological problems facing daughters of women with breast cancer*. Report to the British Psychosocial Oncology Group Annual Conference, December.

Wilkinson, S. (1991) Factors which influence how nurses communicate with cancer patients. *Journal of Advanced Nursing*, **16**(6), 677–89.

Wilkinson, S., Maguire, G.P. and Tait, A. (1988) Life after breast cancer. *Nursing Times*, **84**(40), 34–7.

Wilson, R., Hart, A. and Daws, P. (1988) Mastectomy or conservation: the patient's choice. *British Medical Journal*, **297**, 1167–9.

Wing, J., Cooper, J. and Sartorious, N. (1974) *Measurement and classification of psychiatric symptoms*, Cambridge University Press, Cambridge.

Yasco, J. (1983) Variables which predict burn out experienced by oncology clinical nurse specialists. *Cancer Nursing*, **6**(2), 109–16.

Zigmund, A. and Snaith, R. (1983) The hospital anxiety and depression scale. *Acta Psychiatrica Scandinavia*, **67**, 361–70.

FURTHER READING

Fallowfield, L. and Clark, A. (1991) *Breast Cancer*, Tavistock and Routledge, London.

Faulder, D. (1992) *Always a woman. A practical guide to living with breast surgery*, Thorsons.

Hughes, J. (1987) *Cancer and Emotion. Psychological Preludes and Reactions to Cancer*, John Wiley & Sons, Chichester.

Stoll, B. (1986) *Coping with Cancer Stress*, Martinus Nijhoff, Lancaster.

Tarrier, N. (1987) *Living with breast cancer and mastectomy. Professional self help guide*, Manchester University Press, Manchester.

Tschudin, V. (1992) *Counselling Skills for Nurses*, 3rd edn, Ballière Tindall Ltd., London.

Rehabilitation as an integral part of cancer care | 3

The late Richard Wells

The authors of the various chapters in this book have highlighted some progress in the early detection, treatment and management of people with breast cancer, a trend common to many cancers today. This welcome development places on all health care providers a responsibility to ensure that the quality of life and functioning of the patients and those close to them forms an integral part of their caring strategies, and that we look beyond the tumour and its treatment to address those issues that will enable the individual to return to a useful and fulfilled life. Too often in the past we have failed to do this, failed to institute appropriate initiatives to ensure that the rehabilitation needs of the individual are met. So many people in cancer care assume that rehabilitation will happen as if by magic, when in reality it requires extremely careful planning and a high level of expertise.

There is a great deal of statistical evidence (Cancer Research Campaign, 1982) to demonstrate improved survival for many people with cancer. Overall, the five-year survival rate for all cancers in all age groups is over 35% and constantly improving, and for many of the cancers seen in the young and middle-aged, five-year survival is over 50%. This is much better than that for many chronic illnesses, and it is predicted that by the first decade of the 21st century survival rates will be in the region of 67% (American Cancer Society, 1981). Thus people with cancer will live longer, creating a new type of health care consumer – the cancer survivor.

Cancer careers are frequently marked by exacerbations and remissions and this is especially the case for those with breast cancer. It is therefore most important that health care providers view breast cancer not as an acute illness event, but as a chronic episodic condition, and that they understand the implications of living with the condition and the sequelae of the treatments involved in achieving control of the disease.

Although rehabilitation is a fairly new concept in cancer care, the philosophy applied to other conditions has been espoused for many years; in the 17th century Gasper Tagliacozzi wrote:

We restore, repair and make whole those parts which nature has given and fortune has taken away. Not so much that they may delight the eye, but that they may buoy the spirit and help the mind of those afflicted.

The Concise Oxford Dictionary is less romantic in its definition of rehabilitation: 'to restore privileges, reputation, or proper condition; restore to effectiveness or normal life by proper training', adding in parethesis 'especially after imprisonment or illness'. This is an apposite description for many people with cancer (and those close to them) who may be experiencing something not too far removed from a form of imprisonment.

Concepts of rehabilitation must address the issues surrounding quality of life, defined as a combination of personal satisfaction, emotional status, general health, economic status, previous knowledge, comparison with others, performance ability and self-esteem. In short, the possession of those resources necessary to satisfy the needs of the individual, his or her wants and desires, and an ability to participate in those activities that enhance personal development, self-actualization and allow an acceptable comparison between oneself and others.

Breast cancer is a disease of families as much as it is a disease of individuals. In addition to its affect on many organs and systems of the body, many observers have described the effects of cancer on the social, psychological and cultural functioning of the individual and those close to him or her. These include: loss of confidence, fear of death or disability, fear of becoming an invalid or being overwhelmed by further disease spread. The literature shows that such individuals have great difficulty in adjusting to their condition and in reintegrating into normal life following diagnosis and treatment. Such fears and difficulties are often exacerbated by the negative attitudes towards cancer shared by the public and health care professionals alike (Naysmith *et al.*, 1983; Von Eschenbach and Schover, 1984).

Various studies have highlighted the physical and psychological sequelae of breast cancer. These range from post-treatment functional difficulties and nutritional problems, to difficulties with prostheses, altered body image and psychological disturbance, all of which, for a significant number of people, still exist many years after treatment (Rosillo and Graham, 1972; Greer, Morris and Pettingale, 1979; Heinrich, Greer and Morey, 1987).

THE OBSTACLES TO EFFECTIVE REHABILITATION

There are many obstacles mitigating against effective rehabilitation of the person with breast cancer, and if progress is to be made in this critical area of care these problems must be highlighted and dealt with.

A visit to most hospitals treating cancer patients in the West will reveal groups of dedicated health care professionals offering a wide variety of cancer services; however, most of the rehabilitation specialists will be working in isolation in departments scattered throughout the hospital, and constraints of time, work-load and distance will prevent them from coming together to address the total rehabilitation needs of any individual. As a result the person's deficits are viewed in isolation by each professional group and he or she has to go from department to department to have all his or her needs met.

People often hold unrealistic perceptions of cancer in general and these, combined with the pessimism of some health care providers regarding treatment outcomes, are formidable barriers to appreciating the relevance and value of rehabilitation, as is our failure sometimes to recognize the uniqueness of the patient with cancer and his or her needs.

The assumption that all those who develop cancer will submit rapidly to a painful death is still a widely held view and is a major obstacle to effective rehabilitation, as is the failure to incorporate rehabilitation needs into the plan of care at the time of diagnosis and to involve at that time those disciplines that can effect change. Instead, what appears to happen is that rehabilitation is perceived as something that might occur when the medical disciplines have 'finished' with the patient; for many people this may be too late, condemning them to an inappropriate and unacceptable life after treatment is ended.

Professional jealousies and hierarchical pecking orders are also a bar to rehabilitation: one discipline seeking to dominate all the others seriously impedes a multidisciplinary approach to care, and demonstrates a lack of understanding of the function and purpose of other team members and a failure to appreciate the vital contribution that each can make to the well-being of the patient. Osler reminds us that it is more important to know who has the disease rather than what disease he or she has. All too often we allow the disease to mask the individual and lose sight of the fact that he or she needs attention to many things other than the disease.

The dearth of research demonstrating the value of rehabilitation interventions in the care of people with cancer leads to scepticism on the part of some health care providers. This is changing, however, and several studies by various disciplines are in progress, assessing the benefits of a service that begins at diagnosis and continues throughout the treatment process, demonstrating that early interventions minimize the sequelae of treatment and enhance the quality of life for the individual.

A review of rehabilitation practice for patients following three of the major causes of mortality –stroke, coronary infarct and cancer – reveals a degree of irrationality in the way we view outcomes for the chronically ill.

Rehabilitation strategies following stroke and coronary infarct are vigorous, well co-ordinated and ongoing, despite the fact that 50% of those who suffer a stroke will not survive one year, and 30% of those suffering a coronary infarct will not survive their convalescence period. Comparing these statistics with those of cancer survivorship calls into question the gloomy perceptions of cancer and highlights the need for a rethinking of attitudes towards rehabilitation in cancer care.

REHABILITATION FOR WHOM?

Dietz (1981) enumerates four rehabilitation stages in the care of the person with cancer. These are:

1. Preventative
2. Restorative
3. Supportive ⌐
4. Palliative

The preventative stage begins at diagnosis and is aimed at preventing or minimizing the effects of the disease or its treatment. If there are no residual disfigurements or disabilities people may require few physical services and what is usually most needed are good counselling interventions to enable them to resocialize and break away from their cancer career and sickness role; this latter may have been assumed by them or been thrust upon them. This is also a useful time for the introduction of health promotion strategies to modify potentially harmful behaviours and help improve overall health status.

The restorative stage is the remedying of those disabilities that cannot be avoided in the attempts to eradicate the malignancy. Such patients will often require intensive physical, psychological and social rehabilitation in order to restore to them some meaning for being and reunite them with those things that made life worth living before they became ill.

The supportive stage follows on from the restorative stage and provides care, assistance and support for those having ongoing adaptation problems and those receiving treatment for active disease, usually as a result of secondary occurrence.

The palliative stage offers rehabilitation for those whose treatment has failed or who have relapsed following an initial success. For too many people in palliative care the time between cessation of treatment and death can be long, lonely, unfulfilled and a wasted opportunity, especially when they are surrounded by caring individuals who should assess and meet rehabilitation needs. There is much that can be achieved at this time, and the task is to ensure optimum restoration of function to allow the individual to return to home, work and social interaction, experiencing a good quality of life surrounded by friends or loved ones. Often this does not happen because we fail to appreciate that palliative care is about living, not about dying.

These stages of rehabilitation are applicable to most malignances whatever the age of the patient. The needs of the elderly with cancer are frequently neglected in terms of treatment and rehabilitation, perhaps because they are often perceived as coming towards the end of their natural life, revealing fixed and false perceptions of old age on the part of the health professionals concerned who base their judgements on chronological age rather than the individual.

The number of elderly people is constantly increasing and will provide a significant challenge to cancer services in the future. More than 25% of the population of Western Europe is currently over 70 years of age. There are over 10 million elderly people in the UK at present, and the most rapidly increasing group in the populations of the developed countries are those over 85 years of age. Epidemiological evidence (Cancer Research Campaign, 1982) indicates that cancer has a mean age of onset of around 67.5 years of age.

The literature (Dietz, 1981; Gunn, 1984) demonstrates well that access to clinical trials, aggressive but effective treatments and care based on restoration to as fulfilling a life as possible is not offered to many elderly people because of their age. In the past caring for the elderly has not been viewed as a priority by the majority of health care professionals; cancer in this group is often poorly understood and, some claim, inadequately treated. Caring for the elderly in whatever setting is perceived as an unexciting and unpopular option. As this group will comprise the majority of people seeking cancer care in the future such attitudes are in urgent need of review.

APPROACHES TO REHABILITATION

Cancer is the second largest cause of mortality in the UK and one of the greatest consumers of the health care budget. Breast cancer is the leading malignancy in women, accounting for 20% of all female cancers. Treatments are frequently expensive, arduous and time-consuming and afterwards the individual has a right to believe it has been worthwhile and that she can resume the life and lifestyle she enjoyed before.

Mullen (1984) described a broad-based approach to cancer care which embraces the philosophy of rehabilitation:

> The challenge in overcoming cancer is not only to find therapies that will prevent or arrest the disease quickly, but also to map out the middle ground of survivorship and minimise its medical and social hazards.

Comprehensive cancer centres in the future will need to rethink their strategies in managing the effects of cancer. Combined multidisciplinary approaches will be needed in which the individual with cancer is perceived as the most important member of the team. To facilitate effective communication, interaction and rehabilitation teams should be located in close geographic proximity to each other in designated rehabilitation departments. Membership of the team should be as wide as possible and should reflect the expertise necssary to meet the actual and potential needs of those receiving treatment for cancer. As well as the patient the team could include:

- Physiotherapists
- Occupational therapists
- Dietitians
- Speech therapists
- Appliance fitters
- Dental hygienists
- Music therapists
- Education/information supportive therapists
- Nurses
- Clinical nurse specialists
- Chaplains
- Doctors
- Chiropodists
- Art therapists
- Diversional therapists

This list is by no means exhaustive and can be adapted to reflect local needs or cancer specialties. To ensure that access to rehabilitation is effective, the team should ideally accept referrals from all health care disciplines and self-referral by individuals.

Regarding patients with cancer in the same way as other individuals with other chronic diseases helps us to recognize that recovery or cure mean little if the individuals spend the remainder of their lives secluded from society and totally dependent on others. Bringing together a team of rehabilitation specialists facilitates the sharing of information, provides opportunities to improve the academic standing of the various disciplines and enables the acquisition of knowledge to benefit people with cancer in the future.

SUPPORTIVE THERAPIES IN REHABILITATION

It is well known that over 50% of those receiving orthodox cancer therapies also avail themselves of some kind of supportive therapy. The course of breast cancer often being a slow and incidious process, patients with this disease are frequently among this group. Supportive therapy offers the rehabilitation team the opportunity to extend the remit of its service and to offer supportive therapies as quality of life strategies. The dichotomy that exists between bio-medicine and supportive therapies has a long and tortured history. Unsubstantiated claims of cures and remissions have clouded the issues surrounding supportive therapies, many of which are extremely valuable in helping people feel better.

Properly trained rehabilitation specialists can offer a wide range of useful non-invasive therapies to complement the more traditional approaches to restoration, interventions such as massage, aromatherapy, reflexology, relaxation/visualization, humour, art therapy, music and hypnotherapy. Appropriately used these can all enhance feelings of well-being and aid recovery.

CONCLUSION

Rehabilitation offers new opportunities to be adventurous and graft new approaches to care on to established modalities of treatment. Rehabilitation as conceived in this chapter enables research priorities to be identified and pursued, and the setting of appropriate standards and measurement of outcomes for all disciplines working within the team.

In delivering rehabilitation services it is essential to ensure that control remains with or is restored to the patient, so that she can resume leading as normal a life as possible as quickly as possible. To achieve this it will be necessary to develop a rehabilitation model of care that complements and enhances the medical and nursing models, and pays attention to the particular needs of each individual.

Rehabilitation will form the cornerstone of future approaches addressing the holistic needs of the individual with cancer. Rehabilitation is essentially an applied discipline and must be continually concerned with improving the care of those with cancer; improvement implies change and challenge, with the incorporation of new and exciting multidisciplinary approaches to the development of cohesive cancer rehabilitation services. The ultimate aim must be to prove that we can make a difference to the lives of those who seek our help.

The fight against cancer has left many casualties, whom we could and should have served better. We must use the knowledge they gave us to ensure that those who come after are able to live useful and fulfilling lives whether their disease is controlled or not. As we approach the year 2000 it is not acceptable that people with cancer are handicapped not by their disease, but by our inability or reluctance to see them as unique cultural and social beings and introduce them to those strategies that will help them to be completely well.

REFERENCES

American Cancer Society (1981) *Cancer Facts and Figures*, American Cancer Society, New York.

Cancer Research Campaign (1982) Facts on Cancer: Cancer Research Campaign five year survival rates for cancers diagnosed in England and Wales in 1981, Cancer Research Campaign, London.

Dietz, J. (1981) *Rehabilitation Oncology*, Wiley, New York.

Greer, S. and Moorey, S. (1987) Adjuvant psychological therapy for patients with cancer. *European Journal of Surgical Oncology*, **13**, 511–13.

Greer, S., Morris, T. and Pettingale, K.W. (1979) Psychological response to breast cancer – effect on outcome. *Lancet*, ii, 785–7.

Gunn, A.E. (1984) *Cancer Rehabilitation*, Raven Press, New York.

Heinrich, R.L. *et al.* (1983) Progress in treatment of cancer patients, evaluation of rehabilitation needs. *UCLA Cancer Centre Bulletin*, Fall, 8–10.

Mullan, F. (1984) Re-entry; the educational needs of the cancer survivor. *Health Education Quarterly* (supplement), **10**, 88–94.

Naysmith, A. *et al.* (1983) Surviving malignant disease – psychological and family aspects. *British Journal of Hospital Medicine*, **30**(4), 22–7.

Rosillo, R.H. and Graham, W.P. (1972) Long term adjustment of the patient with head and neck cancer following successful treatment. *Journal of Surgical Oncology*, **4**(5–6), 439–46.

Von Eschenbach, A.C. and Schover, E.R. (1984) Sexual Rehabilitation of Cancer Patients, in (1984) *Cancer Rehabilitation* (ed. A.E. Gunn), Raven Press, New York.

Welch McCaffrey, D., Hoffman, B. and Leigh, S. *et al.* (1989) Surviving adult cancers. III, psychosocial implications. *Annals of Internal Psychological Medicine*, **3**, 517–24.

Screening for breast cancer | 4

Trish Cotton

INTRODUCTION

Breast cancer is the cancer with the highest mortality rate among women in the UK. Some 15,000 women die from the disease every year, a severe loss in both economic and human terms. As the cause of the disease is unknown and primary prevention is not possible, researchers have turned their attention to screening and early detection of breast cancer in an attempt to combat it.

This chapter traces the history of screening from the earliest research to the organization of the National British Screening Programme in the UK, the benefits this was expected to secure, and the nurse's role within the programme.

Following the publication of research from several European countries and the USA, the UK government established a working party to examine the benefit of breast screening. Chaired by Professor Sir Patrick Forrest, the committee examined the evidence available and published its findings in 1986. The committee concluded:

> The information, that is already available from the principal overseas studies, demonstrates that screening by mammography can lead to prolongation of life for women aged 50 or over with breast cancer. There is a convincing case on clinical grounds for a change in UK policy on the provision of mammographic facilities and the screening of symptomless women.
>
> *Forrest, 1986*

The government accepted the report in full in 1987 and its recommendations were subsequently implemented. A national breast screening

programme offered a chance to achieve a significant reduction in mortality from breast cancer. It is informative to look at the evidence examined by the committee.

The Health Insurance Plan of New York

This was a large study, conducted over a period exceeding 20 years, that examined the benefits of mammographic screening. A group of 31 000 women aged between 40 and 64 was selected for screening and a similar sized control group was identified. The women in the study group were offered mammographic screening and physical examination annually for four years.

This study demonstrated that mortality was reduced by 30% for up to 10 years in the women invited for breast cancer screening (Table 4.1) and that a significant benefit was maintained for 18 years (Shapiro, 1977; Shapiro *et al.*, 1988). It is notable that this reduction in mortality was achieved with only a 65% acceptance rate. Whether the improvement in survival would have been increased if the acceptance rate had been higher is unclear.

Table 4.1 The Health Insurance Plan Project*: deaths from breast cancer

	After 5 years	*After 9 years*	*After 13 years*
Study group†‡	39	70	116
Control group‡	63	108	148

*Source: Shapiro, 1977; Shapiro *et al.*, 1988.
†Women in this group offered mammography and a physical examination annually for four years.
‡Women in both groups aged 40–64 years.

The Swedish trial

The Two Counties Study in Sweden (Tabar *et al.*, 1981) studied the use of single view mammography every two years for women in their 40s and every three years for older women. At seven-year follow-up the reduction in mortality was 30% for women aged over 50 years.

At 89% the acceptance of invitation to screening in this study was high. Unfortunately, long-term survival was not demonstrated for women under the age of 50 years.

Nijmegen and Utrecht Studies

Although these two Dutch studies were case controlled rather than random-ized, they still provided important evidence. They demonstrated that women who had been screened were about half as likely as unscreened women to die of breast cancer (Verbeek *et al.*, 1984).

Since the Forrest Report a further report, *Breast Cancer Screening: Evidence and Experience since the Forrest Report* has been published by the Department of Health Advisory Committee (Vessey, 1991). It considered the latest research findings, including further results from the Health Insurance Plan, the Swedish Two Counties Study and the Edinburgh randomized trial. This study published its data on mortality rates at seven years in 1990 (Roberts *et al.*, 1990). Mortality was demonstrated to have been reduced by 17%, but this was not statistically significant; mortality was reduced by 20% in women over 50 years of age. When considering these disappointing results, however, one must take into account the poor acceptance rate, which was as low as 47% in some areas. Lower acceptance was associated with poorer socio-economic groups, a fact that should be remembered when planning and implementing future screening programmes.

The Report of The National Health Breast Screening Programme 1991 concluded: 'if 70% of the population accept the invitation to screening, the reduction in mortality will be about 25%'.

The report presents the potential impact of screening, including a definition in 'human' terms which certainly highlights the improvement in mortality more boldly than statistics alone. The report says:

- After 10 years, 1250 deaths from breast cancer are expected to have been prevented in the UK.
- Each woman in whom death is prevented will live about 20 years longer.
- By the year 2000, the screening programme is expected to have prevented about 25% of deaths from breast cancer in the population of women invited for screening.
- By the year 2000, 25 000 life years will be being gained annually in the UK.

Despite the evidence, not everyone is convinced that screening is worthwhile. One opponent of the screening programme is Skrabanek. He contended (Skrabanek, 1988) that the Forrest report ignored 'data that might undermine unrealistic estimates', and that 'published evidence is distorted. Ethical issues are avoided'. He stated that not a single life was saved in the Swedish study and claimed that overdiagnosis would be a major problem that would lead to unnecessary treatments. It could be argued that Skrabanek was high on rhetoric and low on opposing evidence; however, he made a very valid point on the issue of quality. Skrabanek posed the question: 'Can you transfer a highly sophisticated screening programme, developed in specialized breast units, to the real world of the local clinic?' The issue of quality assurance in screening is one of prime importance on which a screening programme will succeed or fail.

The issue of acceptance is a crucial one: the programme is far more likely to succeed if women attend for screening on a regular basis. Lundgren, the pioneer of the single mammograph technique, stated that health care professionals in the UK needed to gain the confidence of those who had no confidence in the health care system. He went as far as to say that the UK would only have a successful screening programme once this issue was addressed.

Thus, while it could be argued that the opponents of screening are not convincing in their arguments, they have identified possible problem areas to do with acceptance and quality assurance that can be worked on to provide the best possible screening programme for the UK.

ORGANIZATION OF THE UK NATIONAL BREAST SCREENING PROGRAMME

The Forrest report suggested a system for screening (Tables 4.2 and 4.3), while acknowledging that local circumstances may dictate differences in practice. The population of 50–64-year-old women was divided into 'basic screening units' (41 150 per unit). The women within this age group are identified from GPs' lists, held by the Family Health Services Authority (FHSA). Women are sent an invitation to attend for screening that specifies an appointment date and time; this method is considered to achieve a higher response rate, and women are encouraged to change the appointment if it is not convenient. Women over the age of 64 who wish to be screened can arrange an appointment through their GP. Screening takes place in either mobile or static units and recall should be every three years.

Table 4.2 Organization of the UK breast screening programme*: targets

WHO?	All women 50–64
WHAT?	Single view mammography
WHERE?	Static or mobile screening units
WHEN?	Every three years

*As recommended by the Forrest report (Forrest, 1986).

Table 4.3 Organization of the UK breast screening programme*: procedure tree

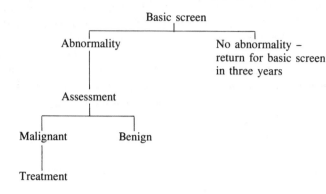

*As recommended by the Forrest report (Forrest, 1986).

Methods of mammography

Mammography is a special X-ray technique, requiring special machinery, that has been developed both to aid diagnosis and to detect impalpable tumours of the breast. The breast is compressed between two plates; compression is essential to produce good quality films. Single view mammography involves taking a mediolateral view of the breast; two view mammography involves a further craniocaudal view. Either can be used in the screening situation.

Many women find that mammography can be rather uncomfortable, so it is wise to provide preparatory warning. After the films are completed, the woman is told that she will be informed of the results within a specified period. The films are then read by a radiologist who considers two factors:

1. Is there an abnormality?
2. What is the likely cause of the abnormality?

The reading of mammograms is a highly specialized skill. Figure 4.3 (a)–(d) shows examples of malignant and benign abnormalities. After reading the films, the radiologist will identify the women who need to come back for further investigation, or assessment. Forrest (1986) estimated that it would be necessary to recall for further assessment up to 10% of women screened in the National Breast Screening Programme.

Assessment

There are likely to be differences in the everyday running of assessment clinics, but what follows is an example of how such a clinic might function. On the woman's arrival the films are reassessed by the radiologist who decides if further mammographic views are required. If so they are taken, and then read by the radiologist. In a few cases, where the recall has been for purely technical reasons, such as the need to take a better film, the woman may be then discharged and advised that she will be recalled for routine screening in three years' time.

If there is an abnormality that requires investigation, the radiologist will consult with the surgeon. The woman will often be seen by both clinicians and a further range of diagnostic investigations may be carried out. This includes clinical examination, ultrasound, fine needle aspiration, sterotactic fine needle aspiration and trucut needle biopsy.

At this stage, a proportion of patients will be found to have a benign condition, for example a cyst may be drained. These women are usually discharged and will be recalled for screening in three years' time. Those who have to await cytology or pathology results will be given an appointment for receiving them. The role of the nurse in the assessment clinic is varied and can include assisting in the clinical situation, explaining the assessment procedure and counselling women who find the whole experience very stressful.

Some women will need an open biopsy for a diagnosis; this is frequently carried out with the aid of guidewire localization of the area to be excised. This procedure will necessitate admission to hospital.

Treatment

By the end of the assessment phase the women will be diagnosed as having a benign or malignant condition. Those who have a benign lesion may simply be recalled for screening three years later. Those who have a malignant lesion will need treatment. The nurse's role is most important at this point.

When a woman presents with symptoms, she has noticed that something could be wrong. However, when a well woman who has experienced no signs or symptoms of a possible breast problem comes for routine screening and is then given a diagnosis of breast cancer, she may well find it especially hard to accept the diagnosis. One can only try to imagine what this feels like. Her initial reaction may be that she is going to die, but it is very likely that a small asymptomatic lesion can be treated and that she will have many good years in front of her. Nevertheless, she will need very skilled counselling to help her come to terms with the diagnosis of cancer and with the change in self-image that may result from her surgical treatment. This is the primary role of the nurse in this pre-treatment phase.

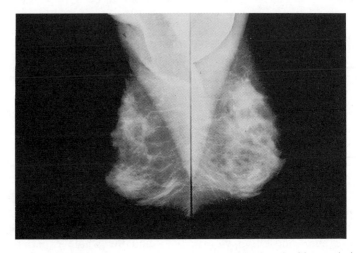

Figure 4.1 Mediolateral oblique view of the breast. Reproduced with permission from Breast-Test Wales.

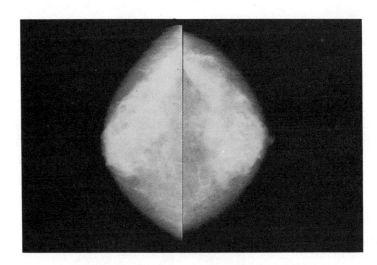

Figure 4.2 Craniocaudal view of the breast. Reproduced with permission from Breast-Test Wales.

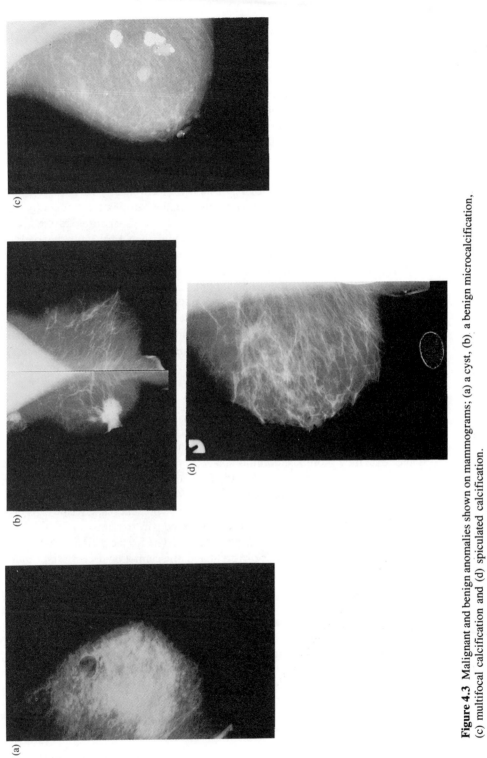

Figure 4.3 Malignant and benign anomalies shown on mammograms; (a) a cyst, (b) a benign microcalcification, (c) multifocal calcification and (d) spiculated calcification.

The psychological effects of breast cancer and treatment are discussed in chapter 2, but we will now examine the approaches that nurses working within breast screening might use.

There is no defined role for nurses at the basic screening test within the guidelines outlined in the Forrest report. It is recommended that a nurse is a member of the multidisciplinary team in the assessment clinic and, while local circumstances may dictate that she be clinically involved in the running of the unit, her primary role is to provide information and support for the women attending.

When women are recalled for assessment they are usually very worried and frightened; they often have no symptoms and their disbelief is frequently obvious. Most women appreciate an explanation of the procedure of assessment and the personnel involved. The nurse should then stay with the patient throughout the procedure. Those who can be told immediately that there is nothing wrong may express their relief in tears; this is just one illustration of the stress these women experience. Those who need to have diagnostic tests, e.g. fine needle aspiration cytology, may have to return for the results. In this situation, after the nurse has answered the woman's questions and given her the opportunity to express her feelings, the nurse should make sure the woman has the telephone number of the clinic and the nurse's name so that she may telephone before returning if she wishes to ask questions or needs support during this anxious time.

Results

When the woman is given the results, whether at the assessment clinic or at a later date they should be communicated in private. Ideally, the surgeon and nurse working together should discuss the results before informing the woman. It is the surgeon's role to break the news gently to the patient that she has breast cancer. Her partner, relative or friend should be present if she wishes. At this stage, if the patient can cope with the information, any treatment options should be discussed with her. Opportunity should be given for the patient to ask questions. While every situation is different and one cannot be prescriptive, there are frequently areas that will require further attention and discussion with the nurse.

- Support
  All patients in this situation will be dismayed by the news. Some will be extremely distressed. The importance and therapeutic value of sitting silently, listening and comforting a distressed patient cannot be over emphasized.
- Many patients will start asking questions about the disase and treatment very soon after being told the news. Verbal information should be given, backed up by written material, such as leaflets. It is important that the information should meet the individual woman's needs, i.e. the information must be appropriate for her.

- If the woman cares for anyone at home or has other responsibilities or problems the appropriate agencies, e.g. a social worker, will need to be contacted to ensure that her admission to hospital can be expedited.

Post-operative care

As with all other women with breast cancer, women diagnosed through breast screening may require the specialist care available from a breast care nurse. Local situations vary and this care is either given by a breast care nurse from the centre where treatment is offered or by the nurse attached to the assessment centre.

It is not only nurses working in the screening situation who are in a position to contribute to the programme's success; all nurses are in a position to promote it. Practice Nurses and those in the primary health care setting are particularly well-placed to give information about the programme and to support those attending for breast screening (Denton, 1989). It is the provision of nursing as much as of radiography, radiology, pathology and surgery that will contribute to and dictate the success or otherwise of the screening programme.

This chapter has concentrated on the role of those working within the screening unit. However, it is vital that other health care professionals, as part of their role as health educators, encourage women in the age group that would benefit from screening to attend for it. There is no doubt that many women's lives could be saved every year if they attended and re-attended for screening. It is vital for all health care professionals to promote screening and to help women to understand the advantages of this programme.

REFERENCES

Denton, S. (1989) Nursing Patients with Breast Cancer, in *Oncology for Nurses and Health Care Professionals*, Volume 3 (ed. R. Tiffany), Harper & Row, Beaconsfield.

Forrest, A.P.M. (1986) *Breast Cancer Screening, Report to the Health Ministers of England, Scotland and Northern Ireland*, London.

Roberts, M.M. *et al.* (1990) Edinburgh trial of screening for breast cancer: mortality at seven years. *Lancet*, **335**, 241–6.

Shapiro, S. (1977) Evidence on screening for breast cancer from a randomised trial. *Cancer*, **39**, 2772–82.

Shapiro, S., Venet, W., Strax, P. and Venet, L. (1988) *Periodic Screening for Breast Cancer: the Health Insurance Plan Project and its sequelae 1963-86*, Johns Hopkins University Press, London.

Skrabanek, P. (1988) The debate over mass mammography in Britain. *British Medical Journal*, **297**, 9701–1.

Tabar, L. and Gad, A. (1981) Screening for breast cancer – the Swedish trial. *American Journal of Radiology*, **138**, 219–22.

Tabar, L. *et al.* (1985) Reduction in mortality from breast cancer after mass screening with mammography. Randomised trial from the Breast Cancer Screening Working Group of the Swedish National Board of Health and Welfare. *Lancet*, **1**, 829–32.

Verbeek, A. *et al.* (1984) Reduction of breast cancer mortality through mass screening with modern mammography. First results of the Nijmegan project. *Lancet*, **1**, 1222–4.

Vessey, M. (1991) *Breast Cancer Screening: Evidence and experience since the Forrest Report*, NHS Breast Screening Programme Publication.

FURTHER READING

Collette, H.J.A. *et al.* (1984) Evaluation of screening for breast cancer in a non-randomised study by means of case controlled study. *Lancet*, **1**, 1224–6.

Watson, M., Denton, S., Baum, M., and Greer, S. (1988) Counselling breast cancer patients – a specialist nurse service. *Counselling Psychology Quarterly*, **1**(1), 25–34.

Surgery for breast cancer | 5

Nicky West and Heather Brown

INTRODUCTION

The majority of treatments for breast cancer involve some form of surgery. This can vary from the smallest excision of the lump, to the – fortunately now rare – extended radical mastectomy. What must be remembered is that all surgery is invasive and carries the risk of side effects. As individuals women may have different anxieties and reactions; similarly, clinicians have differing points of view, ideas and theories. Little in relation to breast cancer and surgery is clear cut or definitive and much is still the subject of debate.

The modern era in surgical treatment of breast cancer dates from the end of the 19th century when Drs William Stewart Halsted and Herbert Willy Meyer reported the results of radical mastectomy. This procedure was used for three-quarters of the 20th century. It was a general belief at this time that breast cancer started as a local disease, extended by direct invasion and lymphatic permeation and was surgically curable until distant metastases occurred. This led to the belief that if tumours were excised quicker and wider the prognosis would be improved. It was not until the end of World War II that the data suggested survival was not improved by extensive surgery (Hardy, 1988).

Surgery can be used in breast cancer to treat primary disease, to support other forms of treatment, to reconstruct the breast following mastectomy, to achieve palliation of local disease, to confirm a diagnosis and the stage of the disease, and finally, but rarely, to treat women considered to be at a 'high risk' of developing breast cancer. It is important to note that other treatments, such as radiotherapy or chemotherapy may be given prior to surgery in order to reduce the size of the tumour, promote management of a fungating lesion or in an effort to control what may be considered to be inflammatory disease.

THE AIMS OF BREAST SURGERY

While it is possibly thought that the reasons for and aims of surgery are identical, it is worthwhile identifying the aims of actually performing such surgery. They fall broadly into two categories: surgery to establish a diagnosis, and surgery as a form of treatment.

Diagnosis

Cells removed in cytology may produce a false negative result or an inconclusive diagnosis. Likewise, not all mammography is conclusive. The only certain method of obtaining a diagnosis may be by surgical intervention, which can then form the foundation for future treatment, etc.

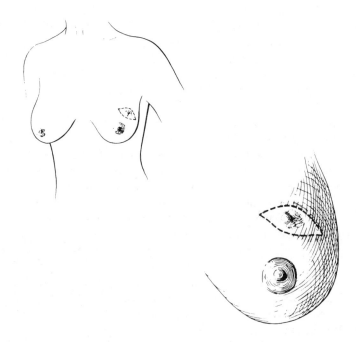

Figure 5.1 Lumpectomy – schematic diagram. Reproduced from Pfeiffer and Mulliken, *Caring for the Patient with Breast Cancer*, published by Reston Publishing Co., 1984.

When surgery is carried out to confirm diagnosis an **incisional biopsy** can be performed. This involves removing part of the tumour for analysis. An **excisional biopsy** involves the removal of all clinically suspicious tissue without paying attention to any margins. This may also sometimes be referred to as a lumpectomy (Figure 5.1).

Treatment

The extended radical mastectomy

This operation involves the removal of the entire breast, the underlying pectoral fascia and pectoral muscles, the ipsilateral axillary nodes and the internal mammary nodes. This operation requires intraplural dissection with removal of a portion of the sternum and ribs.

Sanhani (Sanhani and Tobis, 1986) stated 'There is little doubt that excellent results, in terms of freedom from local recurrence, are achieved by radical mastectomy'. However, today with the further knowledge that it is metastatic disease that patients die from and not uncontrolled local disease, this procedure is very rarely undertaken. In general less extensive surgery is preferred.

Radical mastectomy

This consists of the removal of the entire breast, the underlying pectoral fascia, pectoralis minor and pectoralis major muscles, including the ipsilateral axillary contents *en bloc*. Again, this surgical procedure is rarely undertaken today.

Modified radical mastectomy

There are two types of modified radical mastectomy, the Patey and the Madden operations. The Patey operation involves removing the breast, the pectoral fascia is dissected from the pectoral muscles and the pectoralis minor muscle is either divided or removed. The pectoralis major muscle remains intact. The contents of the axilla are dissected and cleared (Figure 5.2).

The modified radical mastectomy as described by Madden does not involve resection of the pectoralis minor muscle. All patients with operable breast cancer are usually considered to be suitable candidates for this operation as long as the tumour is not fixed to the pectoralis major muscle.

Operative Therapy

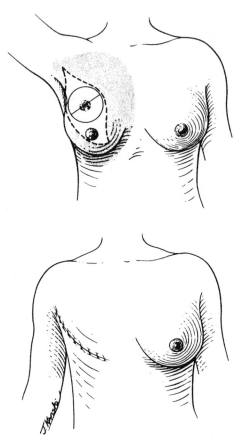

Figure 5.2 Modified radical mastectomy (Patey's operation – schematic diagram. Reproduced from Pfeiffer and Mulliken, *Caring for the Patient with Breast Cancer*, published by Reston Publishing Co., 1984.

Simple mastectomy

This involves removal of the entire breast (Figure 5.3), including the nipple areolar complex, without axillary node dissection or removal of the pectoral muscles. Occasionally one or more nodes may be sampled.

Axillary dissection

The optimal extent of axillary dissection is not clear and opinion differs among surgeons. Dissection can range from sampling (the removal of a node or nodes

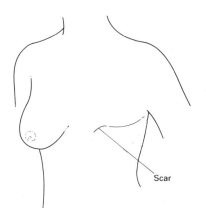

Figure 5.3 Simple mastectomy.

without definition of precise anatomic boundaries) to full dissection of the contents of the axilla up to its apex.

Some believe that the advantages of complete axillary dissection include the fact that it provides prognostic information, helps determine and plan any further treatment, and that this procedure in itself provides a reliable treatment of the axilla.

Palliative surgery

A major consideration when treating women with breast cancer is achieving control of any 'local' disease, i.e. disease within the breast. Where there are distressing fungating lesions or inflammatory carcinomas, surgery can be of assistance to relieve symptoms. Such surgery, however, is usually second or third choice after radiation or chemotherapy. The procedure is not curative, but the aim of the surgery is to enhance quality of life.

Prior to any surgical treatment a full assessment of the patient's breast cancer is generally made. This examination includes an assessment of the size of the breast cancer and the extent of the disease within the breast; the stage of the disease, including examination of the axillary and supraclavicular nodes; and any evidence of distant metastases – investigations such as liver function tests, chest X-ray, bone scan and live ultrasound may also be employed to ascertain this.

Conservative surgery

Although there are still some surgeons who recommend a mastectomy, many are now offering women a choice. Wide local excision followed by radiotherapy has been found to be as effective in terms of overall survival as a mastectomy for women with stage I and II breast cancer. Furthermore, Fisher *et al.* (1989) demonstrated that women who did not receive radiotherapy following conservative therapy had higher local recurrence rates (30%) compared with those who had received radiotherapy (5%). Conservative surgery may be undertaken by performing a local excision, i.e. removal of the tumour together with a margin of microscopically normal tissue, or a quadrantectomy/segmentectomy, i.e. *en bloc* dissection of the tumour within a quadrant of the breast together with underlying tissue (Figure 5.4). Again, the aim is to remove a margin of microscopically normal tissue from around the tumour.

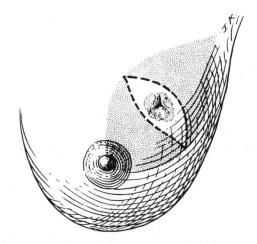

Figure 5.4 Quadrantectomy/segmentectomy – schematic diagram. Reproduced from Pfeiffer and Mulliken, *Caring for the Patient with Breast Cancer*, published by Reston Publishing Co., 1984.

Although the ideal treatment of breast cancer would seem to be breast conservation, many women do still choose to have a mastectomy. Cotton *et al.* (1991) demonstrated that half the patients included in a study chose mastectomy as opposed to wide local excision, and that younger patients were more likely to choose conservation.

Furthermore, it should not be assumed that women choosing conservation suffer any less from anxiety and depression than those undergoing mastectomy. In 1986 Fallowfield (1986) found no difference in terms of anxiety, depression and sexual function between women having conservation therapy and those having mastectomy. In 1990 she and her co-workers

(Fallowfield et al., 1990) found that women whose surgeons offered a choice showed less depression than those treated by surgeons who offered no choice.

Patient choice and the involvement of women in the decision-making process is a significant improvement in breast cancer treatment. Knobf (1990) found that women offered a choice adjust well overall and are less likely to be concerned about recurrence.

It should be noted, however, that not all women are suitable candidates for breast conservation and therefore a choice of surgery may not be indicated. Factors governing such decisions include the size of the cancer, the proximity of the cancer in the breast and the presence of multifocal disease. It is, however, fair to say that breast conservation is a safe and acceptable option for many women requiring surgery.

The overall aims of surgery for breast cancer are to eradicate the primary lesion, achieve an acceptable cosmetic result, minimize the chance of local recurrence and contribute to achieving a good quality of life.

NURSING CARE

For many women, breast surgery may engender a major alteration in body image, leading to considerable psychological morbidity.

Nursing has a vital role to play as part of the multidisciplinary approach in the management of breast cancer, supporting patients from diagnosis through to recovery. Studies have demonstrated that the involvement of specialist nurses from diagnosis may limit the psychological morbidity experienced by patients as a result of earlier onward referral (Chapter 2). (Maguire et al., 1983; Watson et al., 1986).

The giving of information pre-operatively can do much to reduce anxiety levels in patients undergoing investigations and treatment (Hayward, 1975; Boore, 1978), and breast cancer patients are no exception. Wilson-Barnett and Fordham demonstrated that pre-operative assessment and information giving lead to improved post-operative recovery. Although too much information will confuse the patient, especially at the first meeting, often because of the shock experienced when bad news is given, it is nevertheless important to give some information about the proposed treatment.

Women with breast cancer are usually faced with two main problems: the threat to their femininity and body image with all the inherent implications; and the fear of a life-threatening disease. Careful assessment of the patient's needs, fears, anxieties and priorities is therefore essential. It is important to document this in order to reflect back on progress and set realistic objectives and goals for each individual. Many specialist nurses use a standard assessment form, such as the one introduced by Maguire.

Information and support may be offered by a specialist nurse to patients and their families from diagnosis throughout treatment, and many of these nurses see patients in the privacy of their own homes where they may feel more relaxed and more able to ask questions. If a choice of treatment is available to the patient the options may be discussed with her and her family in order to facilitate her making an informed decision.

Breast reconstruction may be offered or discussed at the time of the diagnosis and planning of initial treatment for women undergoing mastectomy. Photographs of the results of such surgery may be shown to patients so they can form realistic expectations of it. In addition there are now many women volunteers who will agree to talk to and show patients considering breast reconstruction their own breast reconstruction.

Post-operative nursing care

Following surgery for breast conservation or mastectomy, patients usually return to the ward with two drainage tubes in place, one placed medially and one laterally. Many patients have undergone some form of axillary dissection and drainage of this area facilitates healing and assists in the prevention of infection.

The wound drains should be checked for patency and amount of drainage, initially every quarter of an hour and then, if satisfactory, every hour for 24 hours, and thereafter at least twice daily. The drainage bags or bottles should be changed and the amount and nature of the drainage accurately recorded once a day, although it may be necessary to change the bags or bottles more frequently if output is high.

Following axillary clearance, seroma formation requiring aspiration may occur in a number of patients (Aitken *et al.*, 1984); it is therefore essential that the drain output is accurately recorded so that it is not removed before necessary. It is also very important to explain to patients why the drain may be in place for a long time. The drain site is a particularly vulnerable area to infection and the use of aseptic technique when dealing with it such as changing dressings, is therefore imperative.

When the amount of drainage over 24 hours is less than 50 ml the wound drain is usually removed. Prior to this some form of analgesia should be offered. Some units have a policy of offering Entonox gas before removing drains.

Some patients may be discharged home with an axillary drain in place, and Holcombe *et al.* (1993) recently conducted a small pilot study looking at this practice. They concluded that it is a safe and feasible option that is liked by many patients and offers considerable resource savings.

Dressings to the site of operation should facilitate mobilization of the arm so that exercises may be begun immediately. Initially post-operative, it is useful to elevate the patient's arm on pillows. This gives comfort and assists the drainage. As the patient mobilizes, she should be encouraged to move her shoulder at least three times a day, covering the full range of recommended exercises. The patient should also be instructed on how to move her arm and hand, and the limb should be observed by staff at regular intervals for colour, possible swelling, and mobility. Exercises should be appropriate for the patient's physical condition, and analgesia may initially be offered prior to any arm exercise as this can assist flexibility as well as removing any potential discomfort.

While in hospital the unaffected arm should be used for blood pressure recordings and injections to reduce any risk of infection and, ultimately, the possibility of lymphoedema. This is a distressing and painful problem that may cause considerable disability. Williams (1992) reports a high incidence of lymphoedema following axillary clearance, and nursing intervention to reduce the risk of it occurring is therefore very helpful.

Finally, patients should be advised about the ongoing care of their arm after discharge, e.g. to avoid cuts, burns and insect bites. If the removal of axillary hair is desired the patient should be advised to use an electric razor to avoid skin puncture and thus possible infection; over-exposure to the sun is not recommended. The arm should be used in everyday activities, but lifting and carrying heavy shopping and luggage should not be undertaken using the affected arm.

Patients should not be coerced into looking at their breast wound. Asepsis should be maintained at all dressing changes and although the wound should be observed for signs of infection and swelling, it is becoming increasingly popular to leave the dressing intact for a number of days if the patient's temperature is normal and the dressing is clean. When the patient is ready to observe her scar site, her husband or partner can be present if she wishes. The patient should be encouraged to look at the scar gradually, and it is therefore useful to suggest she uses a small hand mirror or looks down at the wound before taking a look in a full-length mirror.

As soon as the vacuum drains are removed the patient should be fitted with a temporary prosthesis. Before discharge home she should be given information about how to obtain a permanent prosthesis. Information should also be available regarding bras that are suitable and, most importantly, comfortable to wear immediately following breast surgery.

Throughout treatment women should be encouraged to talk about any fears and anxieties they may have, but care should always be taken not to invade personal privacy. Time and privacy should be made available for discussion, and careful assessment should be made throughout treatment to facilitate early detection of any problems. If a specialist nurse is involved in care she may continue to visit the patient in the community, liaising and referring to other members of the multidisciplinary team as necessary thereby ensuring continuity of care. However, this should be carried out on a very limited basis to prevent overdependence, and when it ceases a contact telephone number may be given to the patient by the specialist nurse together with an invitation to her to telephone if she wants to.

Breast cancer and its treatment can cause a whole plethora of problems both physically and psychologically. Maguire *et al.* (1973) demonstrated that up to one year post-operatively 25% of patients required treatment for anxiety or depression, and Fallowfield (1986) demonstrated high levels of anxiety and depressive illness in 38% of patients undergoing conservative breast surgery.

Surgery is frequently one of the treatments of choice in the management of breast cancer. Problems generated by surgery require identification both by the nursing staff and the other disciplines involved in the care. Nursing intervention with regard to the giving of information, physical care and ongoing emotional support can do much to ameliorate both the physical and psychological problems that patients so often experience.

SKIN CARE

As soon as sutures have been removed, normally around 10 days post-operatively, patients are encouraged to bath and shower in the normal way. Bathing and showering are not discouraged in the initial post-operative period, but care must be taken to keep the wound and any dressing dry. Once the wound is totally healed moisturising cream can be massaged into the wound and under the arm. Those with sensitive skin are advised to use non-perfumed cream.

Deodorant can be used as soon as sutures are removed and wounds healed, as many bath oils or bath salts when taking a bath. Patients should be reassured that their wound may feel hard along the scar site as a result of the formation of scar tissue following surgery, but that it will eventually become soft as the wound heals.

Patients may be informed that this initial nodularity will resolve, but they should be made aware that they must report any skin erythema or nodules occurring on the skin over the chest wall or breast as these might be an indication of recurrent local disease. Such information is essential for the patient, but it should be given with tact to avoid undue worry.

REFERENCES

Aitken *et al*. (1984) Prevention of seromas following mastectomy and axillary dissection. *Surgical Gynaecology and Obstetrics*, **158**, 327–33.

Boore, J.R.P. (1978) *Prescription for Recovery*, Royal College of Nursing, London.

Cotton, T. *et al*. (1991) A Prospective Study of Patient Choice in the Treatment for Primary Breast Cancer. *European Journal of Surgical Oncology*, **17**, 115–17.

Fallowfield, L.J. (1986) Effects of breast conservation on psychological morbidity associated with diagnosis and treatment of early breast cancer. *British Medical Journal*, **293**, 1331–4.

Fallowfield, L.J. *et. al*. (1990) Psychological outcomes of different treatment policies in women with early breast cancer outside a clinical trial. *British Medical Journal*, **301**, 575–80.

Fisher *et al*. (1989) Eight-year results for a randomized clinical trial comparing total mastectomy and lumpectomy with or without irradiation in the treatment of breast cancer. *New England Journal of Medicine*, **320**(8), 22–8.

Hardy, J.D. (1988) *Hardy's Textbook of Surgery, 2nd edn*, J.B. Lippincott Company, London.

Hayward, J. (1975) *Information a Prescription against Pain*, Royal College of Nursing, London.

Holcombe *et al*. The Satisfaction and savings of early discharge with drain in site following axillary lymphadenectomy in the treatment of breast cancer. (Paper awaiting publication).

Knobf, T. (1990) Early stage breast cancer: the options. *American Journal of Nursing*, November, 28–30.

Maguire, P. *et al*. (1973) Psychiatric Problems in the first year after mastectomy. *British Medical Journal*, **1**(6118), 963–5.

Maguire, P. (1975) The psychological and social consequences of breast cancer. *Nursing Mirror*, Volume **140**(14), 54–8.

Maguire, P. *et al*. (1983) The effects of counselling on psychiatric disability and social recovery after mastectomy. *Clinical Oncology*, **9**, 319–24.

Sanhani, R. and Tobias, J. (1986) *Cancer and its Management*. Blackwell Scientific Publications, Oxford.

Watson *et al*. (1988) Counselling breast cancer patients – a specialist nurse service. *Counselling Psychology* **1**(1).

Williams, A.E. (1992) Management of lymphoedema – a community-based approach. *British Journal of Nursing*, **1**(8), 383–7.

Wilson-Barnett, J. and Fordham, M. (1982) *Recovery from Illness*, John Wiley & Sons, Chichester.

FURTHER READING

Demoulin, D. (1989) *A Short History of Breast Cancer*, Kluwer Academic Publishers, Dordrecht, The Netherlands.

Devita *et al.* (1989) *Cancer: Principles and Practice of Oncology*, 3rd edn, J.B. Lippincott Company, Philadelphia.

Radiotherapy for breast cancer

6

Gill Oliver

INTRODUCTION

Radiation has been used therapeutically for some 90 years, a history only slightly shorter than that of X-rays. Over the years it has been increasingly used for treating breast cancer, as evidence has accumulated to show that extensive and mutilating surgery offers little advantage in terms of survival or cure rate (Beckman, 1989).

Despite attempts to raise awareness of the actions and effects of this form of treatment, it frequently remains as something to be feared by those it is prescribed for. Misunderstandings and old wives' tales are still circulated, and credence given to myths and half-truths (Eardley, 1986).

Radiotherapy is prescribed almost exclusively for malignant disease, and so the individual not only has to come to terms with a diagnosis of cancer, but she must also contend with treatment that may be little understood by the professionals, that she herself does not understand, that may last for several weeks, and that may itself produce side-effects that appear worse than the original disease. Elderly people, in particular, may recall stories of radiation accidents, atomic bombs and severe and catastrophic after-effects. The treatment seems to be linked with contamination and patients fear for the safety of their loved ones. Younger people tend to see radiation therapy in terms of mutilation, hair-loss, altered function, loss of quality of life and an inability to continue a normal social existence (Cochrane and Szareweski, 1989).

Effective, efficient care for anyone undergoing radiation therapy depends on initial and continuing assessment, and the benefits of accurate and comprehensible information, given at the correct time, are well documented

(Hayward, 1975; Boore, 1979). Only if the needs of the individual are correctly identified will optimum care be provided; a patient with an understanding of physics may be reassured by factual information about treatment and how it is given, whereas another may be more concerned about the possible changes to her lifestyle during and after treatment (Marks-Maran and Pope, 1985).

Many of the 24 000 women who are diagnosed with breast cancer every year will be treated with one or another form of radiation therapy during the course of their disease (Holmes, 1988). For a large number this will be part of the primary therapy – in conjunction with surgery, for example. Many other women will achieve an enhanced quality of life when radiotherapy is used in a palliative way to control symptoms of advanced disease or, for example, to prevent the development of pathological fractures caused by metastatic deposits in bone.

If women with breast cancer are to receive the care and support that is their right, those providing that care must work from a sound knowledge base. It is not easy to care adequately for a woman having, for example, a five-week course of radical radiotherapy for breast cancer, without having an understanding of the treatment modality. This understanding must include the aims and objectives of therapy, the possible side-effects and the potential hazards. This chapter aims to provide that information, explaining the basic principles underlying radiation therapy, and the effects that this form of treatment may have on the patient's physical and emotional well-being, and on her family and colleagues, too.

In the early years of this century, when radiation therapy was in its infancy, the dangers associated with its use were little understood. Radiation is potentially carcinogenic and there is evidence of skin cancers and other radiation-induced tumours occuring in radiologists working at that time (Duchesne and Horwich, 1988).

Radiation can be machine-made (X-rays, for example, from a linear accelerator), man-made (rendering a substance such as cobalt radioactive in a cyclotron or atomic reactor) or naturally occuring (radium, for example).

Ionizing radiation can take two forms: electromagnetic radiation, including X-rays and gamma rays; and particulate radiation, including protons, electrons, neutrons and alpha and beta particles.

A basic understanding of the principles of radiation is essential if carers are to provide patients with high standards and high quality care and support.

RADIATION THERAPY

Ionizing radiation exerts its effects by dislodging one of the circulating electrons from an atom, rendering it unstable. Chemical and biological changes prevent replication and tumour cells are thus depleted, allowing cure or control of the disease. The current state of knowledge does not allow for selective treatment and so damage will also occur to normal cells included in the treated area, giving rise to the much-feared and discussed side-effects.

In a therapeutic situation the maximum tolerated dose of ionizing radiation will be delivered to the precisely defined part of the body where the tumour is situated. Radiation can be delivered to the patient in a variety of ways. Action at a cellular level will be the same in each case, but the equipment, the length of overall treatment time and the restrictions on the individual may vary considerably.

RADIATION MEASUREMENT

The accepted unit of measurement for the energy in a beam of radiation is the roentgen. However, in the use of ionizing radiation in a therapeutic sense it is the energy that is absorbed in tissue that is important. This used to be described as the radiation absorbed dose, which gave rise to the term rad. The accepted term of measurement is now the gray (Gy). One gray is equal to a radiation dose of 1 joule per kilogram, but doses are commonly expressed now in terms of centigray (cGy) – 100th of a gray, which equals one rad. Thus a dose to a tumour of 5000 rads = 5000 cGy.

METHODS OF DELIVERING RADIOTHERAPY

Teletherapy (External beam therapy)

This is by far the most common method of giving radiotherapy for breast cancer. Teletherapy describes the delivery of an accurately determined dose of radiation energy to a specific part of an individual's body from a machine or source that is at a distance (tele = far). It is used in breast cancer as adjuvent treatment following lumpectomy and biopsy, or after simple or radical mastectomy to remove the tumour. It may also be used: to irradiate adjacent node-bearing areas suspected of malignant involvement; for late presentation of disease, to control local fungation and bleeding; to control the symptoms of metastatic spread, for example to brain or bone; very rarely for metastatic spread to the liver.

Brachytherapy

This term describes radiation therapy whose method of delivery is close up to the site of the tumour. The dose of radiation is provided by a radioactive source which may be in the form of wires, needles or pellets. These are implanted into the breast tissue while the patient is under general anaesthetic, or after-loaded into inert tubes that have been previously inserted. After-loading is generally carried out manually or, increasingly commonly, by a remote controlled after-loading device such as the Selectron.

Implanting or inserting a source of radioactivity into body tissues, although not transferring radioactivity to those tissues, does require certain strict precautions to be taken. All activity around the patient must subsequently be carried out within the terms of the *Ionising Radiation Regulations* (HMSO, 1988).

IMPLICATIONS FOR PATIENTS

A significant amount of the fear associated with radiotherapy is founded in the isolation and protection required. The hazards associated with radiation are well known and documented, and strict rules are laid down for safe practice.

The design of linear accelerators and cobalt machines has changed radically over the years, and whereas such machines tended to resemble items of medieval torture, they are now significantly smaller, more streamlined and sophisticated, and are consequently less frightening. However, it is still necessary for the patient to be alone in the treatment room during the few minutes of the treatment, and although she is continuously watched on closed-circuit television and can be heard on an intercom system, the fundamental sense of being cut off is hard to remove completely.

Much of this natural anxiety can be reduced if the patient understands the rationale for being left alone and has had an opportunity to see the department and the machines before her first treatment.

Isolation during treatment may be one part of the problem, isolation from family and friends another. The high capital cost of complex radiotherapy machines means the treatment is available in only a limited number of sites, which in turn means patients may face long periods in hospital when their physical condition does not in fact warrant admission. Sheer distance from home may limit the opportunities for relatives to vist, further increasing the sense of being cut off. High quality care for radiotherapy patients must therefore encompass far more than the identification of specific therapy-related issues.

SAFE PRACTICE WITH RADIATION

There are significant and known hazards associated with radiation, and its use in an ionizing form must be governed by strict codes of practice. Statutory regulations serve to reduce to a minimum the risk to those working with it.

The *Ionising Radiation Regulations* (Health and Safety Executive, 1985) provide the basic principles on which local radiation protection policies are written, and all staff working in areas where this form of treatment is given have a responsibility to themselves, their colleagues and their patients to be aware of that policy and to practise within its authority. *Guidance Notes* (National Radiological Protection Board, 1988) offer an interpretation of the Regulations, and there is also a *Code of Practice* (DHSS, 1972) relating to the medical and dental use of ionizing radiations.

External beam therapy

Treatment machines are sited in protected rooms, the concrete walls of which are sufficiently thick to attenuate the radiation produced when the machine is switched on (only the patient may remain in the room at this time). An 8 MeV linear accelerator, for example, requires 7 ft-thick concrete walls. Entrance to the treatment room is via an interlocked maze entrance incorporating two right angles; like light, radiation cannot turn corners. The walls of the entrance must also contain appropriate shielding material.

Brachytherapy

It is this form of radiation therapy that carries the greatest potential risk to health care providers. The strictest precautions are required and the patient must be nursed in a designated room or bed within a controlled area; the remainder of the ward becomes a supervised area. Warning notices must be displayed; local rules will govern other working practices – for example, the time any individual spends within a controlled area will depend on the amount of radiation involved.

When caring for a patient who has, for example, iridium wires implanted in her breast tissue, there are three watchwords to bear in mind: time, distance and shielding. It is important to remember that radiation, like sunlight, travels in straight lines. It is also helpful to remember that radiation energy decreases in intensity as distance from the source increases, according to the inverse square law. This means that a nurse who doubles his or her distance from a patient with a source *in situ* from 1 m to 2 m will not halve the radiation he or she receives, but reduce it by a quarter.

Other points to remember are:

- Staff may only enter a controlled area according to a written schedule of work.
- Staff and visitors should spend as little time as possible within a controlled area.
- Whenever possible staff should put as much distance as they can between themselves and the source.
- Shielding should be utilized according to local rules and the advice of the physicist. The need for shielding such as wheeled lead screens or lead aprons will depend on the type and energy of the radioactive source in use.

- The widely recognized black and yellow international radiation warning sign must be prominently displayed whenever ionizing radiations are in use, and all staff must be made aware of their responsibilities within the terms of the regulations.

The development of open visiting has meant that many more people now come in to ward areas and departments where brachytherapy is in use; visitors, families, relatives and visiting professionals must be informed of the restrictions and their activity must be monitored. It is usual to control the visits of young children and pregnant women to patients being treated in this way. (Radiation has the potential to cause mutations since it exerts most of its effect via DNA. As a simple rule of thumb, it is helpful to remember that the most significant damage from radiation occurs in cells that are dividing rapidly, e.g. the bone marrow, hair-bearing areas, the mouth and gastro-intestinal tract and, more specifically, the gonads and the developing foetus).

The levels of radiation exposure of staff working in an area where therapeutic radiation is used are constantly monitored by means of a radiation-sensitive film badge worn by each individual. When developed, the photographic film within the badge provides a record of the radiation the wearer has been exposed to during the period under review. Each badge is specifically identified to a named individual.

The practices and policies detailed above are not intended to be a comprehensive list of radiation protection, they simply highlight those areas that relate particularly to the types of treatment prescribed for patients with breast cancer.

RADIOTHERAPY FOR BREAST CANCER

Radiotherapy will be prescribed at some stage for the majority of women who are diagnosed with breast cancer. For some of these women radical radiotherapy will form part of the primary treatment, which will also include local excision, lumpectomy or mastectomy, with the ultimate objective being to cure the disease. Some women, to whom losing a breast is unacceptable, may actively choose radiation therapy as part of their primary treatment.

In the radical treatment of breast cancer there is general agreement that, whenever possible, the breast should be conserved, especially in early stage disease. If this is not possible then the very best cosmetic effect should be assured. This is best achieved by local excision, which may make very little physical change to the breast, coupled with a radical course of radiotherapy (see below).

Radiotherapy is given with the intention of preventing recurrence in the breast after local excision, or to eradicate known or suspected malignant cells in the area. Radical treatment will most usually be given as external beam therapy using a linear accelerator.

Although specific techniques for delivering radiation to a breast cancer may vary slightly from one centre to another, the principle underlying treatment is to irradiate the chest wall and any breast tissue remaining after local excision or partial mastectomy, plus the node-bearing areas in the axilla, supraclavicular fossa and internal mammary chain. The axilla is not generally irradiated if the axillary nodes have been surgically removed.

Sadly, some women still hide their breast disease through fear or shame, and present late with advanced local disease which may include an offensive fungating ulcer, occasionally of gigantic proportions. This stage of disease is inoperable and primary treatment may well be radical radiotherapy. The objective will be palliation rather than cure, aiming to shrink and dry the fungating tumour and restore some of the dignity and quality of life eroded along with the breast tissue.

Radical radiotherapy (external beam)

An essential preliminary to a radical, curative course of external beam therapy is accurate planning, usually undertaken using a simulator, which is a diagnostic X-ray machine linked to an image intensifier. The simulator reproduces the movements possible on the treatment machines so that angles and distances can be directly translated from one to the other. The radiotherapist is able to see the patient and the X-ray image on screen at the same time, and marks are made on the patient's skin that will later be used to ensure that the treatment beam is accurately directed at the precise area required.

The volume of tissue to be irradiated and the number of fields to be used is assessed. In the treatment of breast cancer it is common to use two or more treatment fields, directing the radiation beam at the patient from a number of different angles.

Much planning work is now computerized and calculations involving radiation physics experts ensure that the dose of radiation is delivered to the required tissue volume as uniformly as possible.

During planning, which for complex treatments may take up to half an hour, the position of the patient will be important. Patients must be able to maintain the treatment position without too much discomfort for the duration of treatment. Special arm-rests may be required when breast tumours are treated.

A course of external beam therapy is spread over a number of weeks. The number of treatments or fractions is decided at the planning stage, although adjustments may have to be made as treatment progresses in the light of the individual's response to treatment.

External beam therapy is most often given on a linear accelerator at energies of 5, 8 or 10 MeV. The first treatment is a time of particular concern for the patient and the care and support required are discussed later in this chapter.

During treatment the patient is required to adopt the exact position decided on during the planning session. The exact area to be treated (the target volume) is identified using the planning marks on the patient's skin, and narrow beams of light or laser beams ensure the energy beam is accurately delivered.

For the short time the machine is functioning the patient must be alone. Actual treatment times average just a few minutes each day, but if more than one field is to be treated additional time will be needed to change the position of the patient and the machine.

In some cases, excision of the primary tumour has allowed only a small margin of surrounding normal tissue, or tumour cells may have been found to extend to the surgical margin. It is then usual for a booster dose of radiation to be given to the excision site after completion of the radical course of treatment. This may be achieved by a single small field of electron beam therapy, deep X-ray therapy, or the insertion of iridium wires.

Approximately 25% of breast cancers are hormone-dependent, and in pre-menopausal women a radiation-induced artificial menopause, altering the hormonal status of the patient, may assist effective disease control for many years. A single session of external beam radiotherapy is used, the results being identical to those achieved with surgical oophorectomy. Radio-oophorectomy may, however, preclude the use of pelvic irradiation in the future when its effects could be required to palliate the symptoms of advancing disease. Drug therapy or adjuvent chemotherapy may also be considered.

Radical treatment with brachytherapy

Rather more rarely, a localized breast tumour may be radically treated by the insertion of a number of iridium wires in the breast tissue. This is carried out in theatre with the patient anaesthetized. Radiation is delivered locally at the highest level tolerated by the patient and at a level that is acceptable in the ward environment. Total treatment time is only a few days.

Alternatively, brachytherapy can also be given by first inserting inert tubes into the breast tissue, again under general anaesthetic in theatre. The patient is nursed in a protected room and the radioactive source is loaded into the tubes at a convenient time either manually (which obviously has implications for staff) or by remote control. This latter method is being used increasingly as it allows the maximum dose to be delivered to the patient while reducing the risk of radiation exposure to staff to an almost negligible level. The Selectron system is one example of a remote-controlled after-loading device.

On completion of the prescribed treatment, sources are withdrawn, again either manually or by remote control, and the inert tubes or applicators removed, if necessary under a light general anaesthetic.

Palliative radiotherapy

Breast cancer frequently metastasizes to brain, bone, lung and liver. Depending on their position in the brain, cerebral metastases may cause changes in personality, sight or movement, for example. Irradiation of the whole brain may achieve control of symptoms for a varying period, occasionally allowing the patient to regain some of the lost function.

Metastatic breast cancer in bones, especially in the spine and femur, commonly causes severe pain as the periosteum is invaded by malignant cells. As bone is destroyed, lytic deposits may be seen, giving the potential for vertebral collapse or pathological fracture. Other metastases may be sclerotic, leading to an increased bone density.

Metastasis in the spine, if not treated as a matter of urgency, may progress to compress the spinal cord causing motor and sensory loss, resulting in irreversible paraplegia. Increased osteolysis resulting from metastasis to bone may lead to hypercalcaemia and its associated physiological effects. These are both oncological emergencies and need urgent treatment.

A short course of radiation to bone metastases can produce a dramatic reduction in pain and encourage recalcification, preventing pathological fracture. This limited intervention can make a radical improvement in quality of life. In the presence of metastatic deposits in the femur, for instance, prophylactic surgical pinning may prevent a future fracture.

Unfortunately, aggressive and advanced breast cancer involving recurrence in the breast or chest wall can cause ulceration, fungation and haemorrhage. Providing the patient has not previously had the maximum dose of radiotherapy to the chest wall, a significant degree of palliation can be achieved with a course of external beam therapy, which will stop bleeding, dry ulcers and lessen the disfigurement associated with fungating disease.

Breast cancer metastases are also seen in liver, and a short course of radiotherapy can provide relief from the associated symptoms: principally pain from an engorged and swollen liver; associated nausea and indigestion; and possibly dyspnoea, too, as pressure is exerted on the diaphragm.

Radiation has a major role to play, not only in the radical treatment of breast cancer, but also in the management, control and palliation of chronic and advanced disease. The judicious use of radiotherapy along with surgery, and cytotoxic and hormone therapy can cure or prolong disease-free survial. When cure is not an option, radiotherapy can be used to great advantage to preserve quality of life for the patient to the highest degree possible.

EFFECTS ON THE INDIVIDUAL

The cases below, adapted from the author's own practice, illustrate the different experiences patients can have of radiotherapy.

Case 1

Beryl arrived at the regional radiotherapy centre accompanied by her husband. Living fairly close to the hospital, Beryl knew she would be able to have her treatment as an out-patient, and during her initial consultation with the radiotherapist she had been given the opportunity to ask all sorts of questions and find out exactly what her treatment would entail. She had made contact with the local breast care nurse, and she and her husband had been able to explore some of their anxieties and fears with her. Beryl had been given some leaflets to take away with her that included pictures of treatment machines and simple descriptions of the treatment and its effects.

Case 2

Sandra had had little time to come to terms with her diagnosis having learnt of her cancer only a few days before her admission. She knew little about breast cancer and understood even less about the radiotherapy that had been prescribed for her. She arrived at the hospital alone having left home, 50 miles away, early that morning. She knew it was unlikely that her family would be able to visit her very often during the four weeks of her treatment – they did not have a car, public transport was infrequent and expensive, and there were the children to consider, too.

Earlier sections of this chapter have discussed radiation therapy, the rationale for its use and the ways it can be directed to specific areas of a patient's body. Although not an invasive technique in the accepted sense of the word, the potential effects of such treatment on an individual can be far-reaching, long-lasting and, in some cases, devastating. This applies to a greater or lesser extent to all people with cancer, but to women with breast cancer in particular.

Emotional responses to radiotherapy

Unfortunately, negative attitudes to cancer in general, to breast cancer in particular, and to radiotherapy are common, and it is in this light that a patient arrives for treatment. The amount of advice and information a patient has received before she arrives will vary radically from none at all to a full and open discussion of her disease, its management, treatment and prognosis. Psychological and spiritual reactions to the prospect of treatment have been identified in several studies (Peck and Bolan, 1977; Gyllenskold, 1982). Physical reactions will be discussed later in this section.

A radical course of radiotherapy for breast cancer may last for four weeks or more. A patient who lives close enough to the radiotherapy centre to travel there each day will have the benefit of remaining at home and sleeping in her own bed at night. She will, however, have the additional strain of the daily journey to and from the centre: ambulance transport is not always available, and depending on family and friends to help can strain relationships to breaking point; petrol costs are high and time is precious. Even if the patient continues to feel quite well during treatment, travelling can take up a large proportion of the day, disrupting social activity and family life. Also, out-patients may sometimes feel cut off from the supportive networks available to in-patients and their families.

In-patient treatment has its own problems. A long period away from home can lead a woman to lose her sense of self-worth, her role as mother or wife disappears and, if distance from home means long travelling times, visitors may be infrequent.

The perceptions and attitudes of a woman to her breast cancer will be affected and shaped by the aims and objectives of the treatment she is coming for. For example, a radical course of radiotherapy can be promoted as a very positive intervention aimed at cure or, at the very least, at a long disease-free interval. However, a woman attending for palliative radiotherapy for painful bony metastases may have lived with her breast cancer for many years and be well aware that cure is no longer an option, and that her expectations may be restricted to a reduction in her pain and an improved quality of life. In either case, negative perceptions of radiotherapy create increased and unnecessary levels of anxiety and distress.

Physical and emotional reactions to treatment vary from one individual to another depending on dose, target volume, skin type and the psychological and emotional preparedness of the patient. It is important to consider the effect of treatment on the woman's partner too, and whenver possible both should be involved in discussions and decision-making. For single women, the implications of the disease and its treatment may be the cause of great anxiety, with fears centring around making new relationships and explaining things to new partners.

Physical responses

The breast

The majority of physical effects related to radiotherapy are seen in the area being treated. Radiotherapy to the breast and chest wall means that each beam must first pass through skin, and since the germinal layer of the epidermis contains cells that are rapidly dividing, some reaction may be seen. With the rapid development of modern treatment machines and an enhanced skin-sparing effect, the much-feared 'radiation burns' of the past are rarely seen now. However, a mild erythema, showing as a reddening and irritation in the treatment area, may develop two weeks or so after treatment has begun. In some people, particularly those with sensitive skins, this may develop to dry desquamation, when the skin becomes dry, flaky and irritating.

Radiotherapy is not begun until the scars from any previous surgery have completely healed, but the area around the scar may still be very sensitive. When skin surfaces are opposed, such as beneath the breast and in the axilla, an area of moist desquamation may occur, when the integrity of the skin is lost. A serous exudate may predipose to infection and the area becomes reddened and sore.

When a large area is being treated the oesophagus may be included, and the sensitivity of the lining cells can cause a sore throat and sometimes indigestion. The position in which a woman is treated may be awkward for her, particularly if she has had previous surgery. Stiffness and pain in the shoulder can sometimes be a problem.

Treating a tumour with radiotherapy means that the toxic results of cell breakdown must be excreted from the body by normal metabolic processes. This may lead to feelings of general malaise, lethargy, insomnia and depression. Nausea and vomiting may, though by no means always, be a feature of radiotherapy for breast cancer. Several theories may account for this: stimulation of the chemoreceptor trigger zone in the brain by toxic waste products from cell breakdown, peripheral stimuli from the gastro-intestinal tract, or impulses from the middle ear similar to travel sickness (Holmes, 1988).

These symptoms, in turn, may well affect the patient's appetite, concentration and relationships. The psychosexual responses to a diagnosis of breast cancer and its treatment (discussed in Chapter 2 and 15) add another dimension to the problem.

Areas of metastasis

Areas of the body other than the breast may be treated to control or palliate symptoms of advanced disease, and to enhance quality of life. The psychological and emotional reactions to such treatment will be significant and it is important that the toxic effects of the treatment do not outweigh the benefits to be achieved.

Cerebral irradiation for metastases will always cause hair loss and possibly some skin irritation and flaking. Raised intracranial pressure may give rise to headaches and occasionally fits. Such symptoms are distressing for the patient and often considerably more so for family and friends. The required treatment, diuretics and steroids, may itself give rise to unpleasant symptoms.

Palliative radiotherapy for bone metastases from a breast tumour is usually well tolerated, the short course of radiotherapy producing little in the way of side-effects for the patient. However, in the presence of widespread bone metastases, an upper or lower hemibody field may be prescribed. The size of the treatment field will lead to toxicity and almost certainly nausea and vomiting. The benefit of pain relief outweighs the possible side-effects, which are transitory and should in practice be preventable.

Liver involvement from breast cancer may be t
It is unlikely that overall survival time will be inc
that treatment does not provoke any additional sym
this stage is extremely poor.

Radiotherapy may affect an individual emotionally, psyc
and physically. The extent to which these effects may be
on the patient's own knowledge and perceptions of the treatment pr
her physical condition, and the dose and length of treatment.

The care and support in terms of nursing interventions that these patients rightly expect are detailed in the next section, but it is worth stressing that effective care will never be achieved without accurate assessment of needs by a carer with sufficient knowledge of the treatment modality. Assessment and subsequent care-planning demands the active participation of patient, nurse and family, too, while continuing evaluation will ensure that care is relevant and objectives are being met.

NURSING INTERVENTIONS

The need for psychological and emotional support for radiotherapy patients is equally as great as the need for physical and practical care.

The woman coming for breast cancer radiotherapy may be approaching treatment with a little knowledge or a great deal. She may have had little notice of her appointment, she may have been at home, post-operatively, waiting for her mastectomy scars to heal in the knowledge that her six weeks of radiotherapy loomed ahead. In either case, the woman has had to face a diagnosis of malignancy; her reactions to that and to the prospect of radiotherapy may have left her feeling bewildered and unable to cope.

Effective care must be founded on a comprehensive and accurate assessment of all her needs. She needs the facts about the disease itself, the investigations and planning that may be needed before radiotherapy starts, how treatment will be given and the possible effects it may have. It is not enough just to tell her these facts or hand out a leaflet – the carer must ensure that the messages have been understood. It is always helpful to involve a third party – husband, partner or friend – to assist the woman to recall what has been discussed, and some centres are experimenting with tape recordings of consultations, which patients may take home and replay at their leisure (Hogbin and Fallowfield, 1989).

The rationale for treatment, tests and investigations needs to be explained and, although it may come from the doctor in the first instance, it will invariably require restating and reinforcing. The patient's particular anxieties must be discovered and, as far as possible, allayed. Long-held beliefs, myths and

...rstandings may be deeply rooted, and much time and effort may be ...ed to resolve them.

Effective support will require:

- an appropriately trained, skilled and knowledgable nurse;
- access to such an expert nurse for all breast cancer patients referred for radiotherapy;
- a quiet area of privacy where consultations can take place;
- written or recorded information to back up face to face interviews and conversations.

Nursing interventions must be planned to prevent or minimize the various physical and physiological responses to radiotherapy. Effective and positive outcomes will depend on an accurate assessment of the patient and her problems and a plan of care that demonstrates a problem-solving approach or one that is model-based – for example, activities of daily living and how these may be compromised by disease and its treatment.

Teletherapy

Nursing action is planned to prevent potential skin problems related to the treatment:

- treat skin in the treatment area gently;
- prevent further irritation and inflammation by avoiding perfumes, deodorants, creams, lotions, very hot or very cold water and harsh towels, and warn the patient against tight clothing (e.g. collars and bras);
- suggest the patient wears cotton clothing;
- expose treatment area to fresh air for several periods of 20 minutes to half an hour each day, but avoid exposure to sun or cold wind;
- warn patients that planning marks should not be removed, but may rub off on to clothing and may show above necklines; an old cotton T-shirt can protect top clothes and a scarf may hide obvious marks.

If dry or moist desquamation occurs, symptoms may be lessened by:

- application of baby powder or maize starch to cool skin and reduce irritation (if skin is unbroken);
- application of 1% hydrocortisone cream may reduce inflammation, but may also mask the development of fungal infections; preferences will vary from one centre to another but the application of povidone-iodine or proflavine can be soothing if rather messy;
- application of simple non-adherent dressings to reduce friction between skin surfaces and prevent infection of moist area; this is a particularly important consideration if the patient has pendulous breasts since the inframammary fold is especially vulnerable to this problem.

Interventions to prevent and minimize the systemic effects of radical radiotherapy include:

- the prescription of a period of rest each day, particularly following treatment;
- the prescription of mild night sedation if insomnia is a problem;
- discussion and advice on an acceptable balanced and nutritious diet that will provide sufficient calories and/or referral to a dietician for specialist advice;
- bland foods, milky drinks and frequent oral fluids to counteract dysphagia and indigestion;
- regular inspection of oral mucosa and initiation of oral hygiene routines;
- encourage increased oral liquids, up to 2–3 litres in 24 hours, to encourage excretion of toxic waste products from cell breakdown:
- prescription of humidified air, simple linctus or inhalations if radiotherapy has irritated the bronchial lining.

Nursing interventions may also be indicated in response to physical changes:

- help with simple shoulder exercises so that treatment position can be comfortably maintained; referral to physiotherapist for specialist advice;
- encourage patient to use affected arm, for example when hair-brushing, dressing, etc.;
- compression bandages, arm hosiery and the use of intermittent compression pumps may reduce the discomfort of lymphoedema; referral to a specialist should be made whenever possible;
- stiffness, discomfort and lymphoedema may be minimized by ensuring cushions, pillows, reclining chairs, etc. are used to the best advantage.

Brachytherapy

The nursing role in brachytherapy may include the following interventions in addition to those detailed above:

- factual explanations about restrictions to the patient and her visitors while the sources are in place;
- prevention of infection by regular cleansing of exit and entry points of applicator or source;
- accurate completion of radiation protection documentation.

Nursing interventions when radiotherapy is prescribed as palliation relate almost totally to the problems associated with the disease and its progression. It is important that palliative radiation therapy does not produce any new symptoms or any dramatic local side-effects, or create distressing systemic responses in the patient. The nursing care of advanced disease is discussed elsewhere, but specific radiotherapy-related nursing interventions are considered below.

Cerebral irradiation

- As hair loss occurs patients may like to have their hair cut or head shaved. A hair net can prevent hair falling into food or on to the pillow at night. Some women may require a tremendous amount of support while undergoing this process. It is essential to organize the supply of a wig, if the woman wishes, in advance of the hair loss.
- E45 applied to the scalp will soothe scaly and irritating patches. It is particularly important to pay attention to the areas behind the ears.
- The steroids that may be prescribed to reduce therapy-related cerebral oedema may create an increase in appetite. Advice on and control of diet is necessary with relevant explanations to patient and family.

Irradiation for bone metastases

If spinal cord compression from metastatic disease is suspected or present the therapy prescribed is an emergency intervention and has the potential to cause severe nausea and vomiting. Although this is a palliative course of action, the possibility of side-effects is usually acceptable when balanced against the benefits of preventing further complications from compression and subsquent motor and sensory loss.

Active intervention to prevent nausea and vomiting will also be required prior to hemibody irradiation, again a palliative intervention but one with the potential to improve dramatically the quality of life of the patient concerned.

Nursing interventions must include:

- administration of prescribed anti-emetic medication and evaluation of its effect;
- monitoring of intravenous infusion by which anti-emetic therapy is given;
- assessment of need for additional, complementary methods of managing nausea, such as relaxation, massage or music.

The nature of radiation therapy means that only a few minutes each day are required for treatment. Patients who are being treated as in-patients but who are physically quite well may have a significant amount of 'spare time'.

Nursing care must include:

- assessment of each patient's need for help;
- developing programmes of diversional therapy;
- organizing visits from voluntary and charitable groups who may provide entertainment, quizzes or games sessions;
- liaison with other members of the multiprofessional team;
- liaison with the therapy department to agree treatment times that allow for visits to local shops, theatres, etc.

Nursing interventions for patients with breast cancer having radiotherapy must encompass both theoretical and practical aspects. The importance of accurate assessment of need and the availability and accessability of knowledgable staff cannot be overstated.

SUPPORT SYSTEMS

Breast cancer can be a chronic disease following a course of many years. Radiotherapy may be prescribed at different points during this time, initially as radical treatment and later for disease recurrence and metastases, and palliation of the symptoms of advanced disease.

It is important that facilities are available within the radiotherapy centre for support and counselling. As the woman may move several times from one care setting to another, a comprehensive system of referral should ensure that the necessary information follows the patient and that the key workers in each new setting are familiar with the needs of the patient and the means that have been employed to meet them.

While not all centres will be sufficiently large to include representatives of all the associated professions on the permanent staff, policies must identify ways in which referrals for specific help can be made without delay, for example to a physiotherapist, an occupational therapist, a dietician or a medical social worker.

Within nursing, individuals will develop particular skills and experience, for example in breast care, lymphoedema or the management of fungating wounds. This expertise must be utilized by prompt referral. Where this specialist advice is not immediately available, efforts should be made to identify alternative sources of help.

There are charitable and voluntary organizations with particular relevance to breast cancer patients and self-help and support groups provide a non-threatening environment where patients and families can meet.

National organizations such as Breast Cancer Care (formerly the Breast Care and Mastectomy Association) have local branches throughout the country, and volunteers are available to visit women having breast cancer treatment. Other organizations offering information and advice are listed in Appendix A.

Radiotherapy is one of the principal treatment modalities for breast cancer. Women often come with many preconceived ideas about its delivery, usefulness, effects and dangers. By its nature, radiotherapy must often be given over a period of weeks. Care and support cannot then be narrowly focused on the short time that a woman is actually receiving her treatment. Although this will be important, so too will the implications of treatment for her functioning, lifestyle and relationships. It is to these areas that care must be directed. A quality nursing service for these women will include not only explicit statements about agreed standards of care, but also systems of monitoring and evaluating that care so that all those involved can demonstrate that efficient and effective delivery of care has been achieved.

REFERENCES

Beckman, J. (1989) *Breast Cancer and Psyche*, Ideas International, Odense.

Boore, J. (1979) *Prescription for Recovery*, Royal College of Nursing, London.

Cochrane, J. and Szareweski, A. (1989) *The Breast Book*. Macdonald & Co., London.

Department of Health and Social Security (1972) *Code of practice for the protection of persons against ionizing radiations arising from medical and dental use*, HMSO, London.

Duchesne, G. and Horwich, A. (1988) in *Oncology for Nurses and Health Care Professionals*, Volume 1 (ed. R. Tiffany), Harper and Row, London.

Eardley, A. (1986) Radiotherapy: what do patients need to know? *Nursing Times*, **82**(16), 24–6.

Gyllenskold, K. (1982) Breast Cancer: the psychological effects of the disease and its treatment. *International Journal of Nursing Studies*, **25**(2), 117–24.

Hayward, J. (1975) *Information: a Prescription Against Pain*. Royal College of Nursing, London.

Health and Safety Executive (1985) *The Ionising Radiations Regulations*, no. 1333, HMSO, London.

Hogbin, B. and Fallowfield, L. (1989) Getting it taped: the 'bad-news' consultation with cancer patients. *British Journal of Hospital Medicine*, **14**, April, 330.

Holmes, S. (1988) *Radiotherapy*, Lisa Sainsbury Foundation, Austen Cornish, London.

Marks-Maran, J. and Pope, B. (1985) *Breast Cancer Nursing and Counselling*, Blackwell Scientific Publications, London.

National Radiological Protection Board; Health and Safety Executive (1988) *Guidance notes for the protection of persons against ionising radiations arising from medical and dental use*, HMSO, London.

Peck, A. and Bolan, B. (1977) Emotional reactions to radiation treatment. *Cancer*, **40**(1), 180–4.

FURTHER READING

Copp, K. (1989) in *Oncology for Nurses and Health Care Professionals*, Volume 3, (ed. R. Tiffany) Harper and Row, London.

Oliver, G. (1989) in *Nursing the Patient with Cancer* (ed. V. Tschudin), Prentice Hall, London.

Thomson, L. (1989) *Nursing the Patient with Cancer* (ed. V. Tschudin), Prentice Hall, London.

Chemotherapy for breast cancer

7

Trish Cotton

INTRODUCTION

As one of the major weapons in the battle against cancer, cytotoxic drugs have one of the shortest histories. It was in the early years of this century during a time of war (when so many medical discoveries and innovations have taken place) that the cytotoxic effects of mustard gas were discovered. This led to the development of one of the first drug treatments for cancer – nitrogen mustard. It is only some 50 years since this first compound was isolated, and during the intervening years hundreds of substances have been identified and tested, discarded or retained, until in the mid-1990s there are some 40 or so cytotoxic agents in common use.

Mustard gas caused extensive vomiting in those affected by it, and the nitrogen mustard developed from it was no exception. As more drugs were discovered, so the toxic side effects they engendered came to be perceived as part of the effect of these drugs. 'Chemotherapy' gained the reputation from which it has struggled to escape ever since: in the eyes of the public, cytotoxic chemotherapy is inextricably linked with hair loss, nausea, vomiting and a range of other toxic, debilitating and distressing effects.

CYTOTOXIC DRUG ACTIVITY

Cytotoxic drugs exert their action in a number of different ways, but the end result is always to prevent cell division and thus eradicate or control malignant disease, the rate of cell growth of which is erratic and uncontrolled.

At the same time, cytotoxic agents affect the growth of normal cells, leading to the well-known side-effects that include neutropoenia and alopecia.

CLASSIFICATION OF CYTOTOXIC DRUGS

Cytotoxic drugs can be classified in a number of ways, but one accepted method is to define them according to their activity on the process of cell division. Nitrogen mustard, for example, belongs to a group of drugs known as alkylating agents, which have the ability to cross-link strands of DNA and thus prevent their separation. Methotrexate, another of the early agents, prevents the cell from manufacturing DNA and, by definition, thus belongs to the group known as antimetabolites.

The vinca alkaloids exert their destructive action by preventing the partition of the two strands of DNA. They are known as spindle poisons,

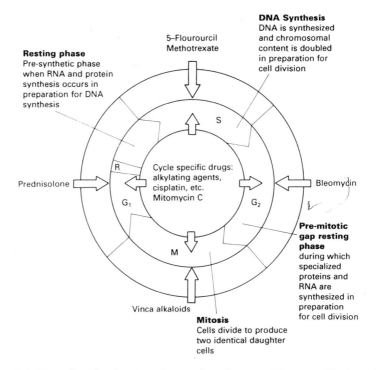

Figure 7.1 The cell cycle, showing where various drugs act. Phase-specific drugs in the outer band act at specific stages of the cell cycle; cycle-specific drugs in the centre act on the cells throughout the cell cycle.

and prevent the spindles that join the two DNA strands from pulling them apart. Another group of drugs acts by interfering with the function of DNA, and these are sometimes referred to as intercalating agents.

In any system there are always some items that fail to fit exactly into any category and cytotoxic drugs are no exception. Some commonly used drugs falling into this category are bleomycin and mitomycin C for example. Figure 7.1 shows where various drugs act.

Cytotoxic agents all have a degree of specificity and, as will be seen later in this chapter, only a relatively small number of drugs are used in the management of breast cancer. Cytotoxic drugs are produced in a range of presentations suitable for oral, intravenous, intrathecal, intra-vesicular, topical, and intra-arterial use. The implications for staff and patients vary considerably, and will be discussed later. It is rare for any preparation other than oral or intravenous agents to be used for patients with breast cancer.

SAFETY OF CYTOTOXIC DRUGS

Cytotoxic drugs are themselves inherently carcinogenic and must be handled with respect. Strict policies and guidelines are required wherever such drugs are used, and it is an absolute requirement that staff are educated, trained and skilled in the wide range of required competencies.

EFFECTS OF CYTOTOXIC DRUGS ON INDIVIDUALS

The effects of cytotoxic agents on individuals are well documented; they affect patients' physical, social, psychological and emotional well-being. The patient with breast cancer, who has already had to face a diagnosis of malignancy, and possible major surgery and the disfiguring effects of mastectomy too, must then come to terms with a lengthy course of drug treatment that affects her well-being, role and self-image. Her ability to work may be compromised, and her roles as mother, wife or lover may be further eroded.

General side-effects

The side-effects of cytotoxic drugs can be subdivided into those that appear immediately, those that appear in a number of hours or days, those that may be seen in months, and long-term effects that are still present many years after treatment.

The most common side-effects of cytotoxic chemotherapy include hair loss, nausea and vomiting. They are the two side-effects most patients fear above all others and they generally believe that they are inevitable. But modern cytotoxic chemotherapy for breast cancer does not necessarily involve hair loss or extreme nausea.

Immediate side-effects

At the time of administration of venous chemotherapy, great care must be taken in siting the cannula and then in observing the infusion site. While extravasation – leakage of the solution into the surrounding tissue – is not truly a side-effect, it can cause such discomfort, pain and trauma to the patient that it must be considered seriously. If extravasation occurs, the patient will complain of pain at the infusion site and it may be severe. The treatment of extravasation has been the subject of some research and little consensus. The advice of drug companies and pharamcists should be sought in formulating a hospital policy for treating this effect of chemotherapy. A serious extravasation can result in necrosis of the surrounding tissues and may require plastic surgery to correct it. Therefore only trained skilled nursing and medical staff should administer chemotherapy.

As the cytotoxic agent travels along the vein, some patients may complain of heat, cold or pain along its route. Some patients experience flushing of the face and/or body, and an abnormal taste and smell is not unusual. Some may suffer general reactions and, rarely, anaphylaxis.

Short-term side-effects

Some patients may experience gastro-intestinal side-effects, such as anorexia, nausea, vomiting, constipation or diarrhoea, in varying degrees and for varying periods. A generalized malaise accompanied by pyrexia for some days may be experienced by some.

Side-effects concerned with the genito-urinary tract may include haematuria and, fairly commonly, discoloured urine, e.g. green discolouration urine after administration of Mitozantrone.

Long-term side-effects

Chemotherapy may cause long-term side-effects; some of the effects of these drugs in the long-term are not fully understood, e.g. amenorrhoea and sterility. Chemotherapy has an effect on the sexuality of any patient, loss of libido may occur along with other side-effects such as headaches, lethargy and depression. The long-term genetic side-effects of chemotherapy are also not fully understood. Animal studies have demonstrated that cytotoxic drugs can cause mutogenic and tetratogenic changes in offspring. Certainly, patients undergoing chemotherapy should be advised of the necessary time delay between completing the course of treatment and conceiving a child.

Bone marrow depression is another potential side-effect, as is alopecia and skin rashes; along with gastro-intestinal upsets, these are probably the most common side-effects. There is also a risk of pulmonary fibrosis, congestive cardiac failure and liver and renal toxicity.

USE OF CHEMOTHERAPY IN BREAST CANCER

Cytotoxic chemotherapy has been commonly used as a treatment for advanced breast cancer; indeed, some members of the public perceive that chemotherapy is only ever used as a last resort. As more research is carried out it is clear, however, that chemotherapy is an appropriate treatment for early breast cancer.

Pre-operative treatment

Chemotherapy can be used before surgery in an attempt to reduce tumour bulk. This is an attempt to reduce the incidence of uncontrolled local disease (a most distressing condition) after surgical treatment. This method of treatment is generally used for women who present with large tumours, since reducing the size of the tumour chemically may make it possible to employ less radical surgery.

Adjuvent treatment

Adjuvent chemotherapy is used after primary surgery to the breast, often in patients with poor prognosis tumours. While hormone manipulation is commonly prescribed for post-menopausal patients, cytotoxic chemotherapy is increasingly being prescribed for pre-menopausal patients with axillary node involvement.

There is evidence that the disease-free interval (i.e. the time from treatment to recurrence) and survival are both improved by the use of chemotherapy. Some studies have shown this benefit more strongly for pre-menopausal patients.

Advanced breast cancer

It must be accepted that cytotoxic chemotherapy used in patients with advanced breast cancer is palliative only. The benefits of such treatment must always outweigh the side-effects and it is important that the patients themselves understand this: it is very sad to see such patients undergoing chemotherapy, which is clearly causing them great distress, in the vain hope of a miraculous cure.

The role of nurses in meeting information needs and ensuring patients have a realistic expectation of the treatment is important, and the multidisciplinary team must work together to ensure continuity of care and full discussion of the disease and treatments.

DRUGS COMMONLY USED IN BREAST CANCER

Many drugs are often given as combination chemotherapy, for example cyclophosphamide, 5 Fluoro-uracil and methotrexate (CMF). The most common are listed in Table 7.1. It is impossible to give an exhaustive list of drugs and possible combinations, however, as knowledge is constantly increasing through research.

Drugs may be installed into cavities within the body in order to limit metastatic spread. In breast cancer, the lung is a common site for metastatic disease and this sometimes results in malignant pleural effusion. One treatment for this is draining and re-expanding the lung, and then installing cytotoxic drugs in the pleural cavity, both as a sclerosing agent to achieve pleurodesis, and as a cytotoxic agent. Bleomycin is commonly used for this purpose.

Meningal secondary deposits in breast cancer are rare, but may be treated by intrathecal administration of the drug methotrexate.

Table 7.1 Cytotoxic drugs commonly used in intravenous therapy for breast cancer

Cyclophosphamide *5 Fluorouracil* *Methotrexate*	*Commonly used in combination*
Epirubicin hydrochloride	Single agent or in combination with above
Adriamycin	Single agent or in combination with above
Mitozantrone Mitomycin C Methotrexate	Single agent or in combination with below

NURSING CARE

Most patients receive chemotherapy in an out-patient clinic. It is vital that nurses are present and that patients have a contact telephone number for specialist advice and help while they are coping at home. Not all patients receiving chemotherapy will suffer badly from side-effects; indeed, it is the aim of nursing care that they should not.

It must be remembered that patients receiving chemotherapy for advanced disease are not only coping with the treatment, but are also likely to be trying to come to terms with the advanced stage of the disease and all its implications. The value of listening to these patients cannot be overestimated – talking things through will help the patient to start to come to terms with her prognosis. She may require help from palliative care specialist nurses or doctors, or, rarely, from a psychiatrist or psychologist, and it is important for nurses to recognize when such a referral is appropriate. Social workers, health visitors and community nurses may also need to be involved, particularly if the patient has responsibilities such as children or an elderly dependent relative. (The psychological aspects of breast cancer are discussed more fully in Chapter 2.)

If patients are nauseated as a result of their chemotherapy, adequate anti-emetics must be prescribed. These can either be given orally or by injection. Oral anti-emetics can be started a day before the chemotherapy is to be given and continued for as many days as is necessary after the treatment. Intravenous anti-emetics can be given at the same time as the chemotherapy, and injections by other routes can be administered at home by community nurses or family doctors as required.

Anti-emetic therapy is vital to help ensure adequate nutrition. For some, vomiting becomes so severe that it can be triggered off by something related to the treatment, such as the sight of the hospital or of the individual who administers the drugs. This is a most difficult problem to solve; strong regular anti-emetics may help, but some patients may need the expertise of a psychiatrist or psychologist to overcome this distressing condition.

The recent introduction of a new group of drugs, 5-HT$_3$ receptor antagonists, has greatly increased the potential to limit and control nausea and vomiting induced by cytotoxic chemotherapy.

Some patients may suffer hair loss and this may range from slight to complete, although it is usually temporary. Patients should be warned that alopecia is possible, and advice should be given to minimize the risk: washing the hair with baby shampoo and conditioning, avoiding heat when drying, and avoiding chemicals such as dyes and perms are helpful suggestions. Patients with long hair may minimize the risk by having their hair cut in a shorter style prior to treatment. When alopecia seems inevitable a wig should be provided as early as possible, if the patient wants one. Other patients may prefer hats or turbans instead.

Attention should also be paid to the patient's skin care as skin reactions may occur. It is advisable for the patient to avoid strong sunlight on the skin. Dry skin should be treated with a simple moisturizer.

Some patients will suffer a form of cystitis due to inflammation of the bladder lining as a result of the cytotoxic therapy. Adequate fluids are essential and vomiting is likely to worsen this symptom. Some cytotoxic drugs will cause discoloration of the urine, it is vital to warn patients as this can be very frightening.

Nurses should, of course, observe patients for signs of toxicity apart from the ones mentioned here. Renal and cardiac toxicity are important, but not commonly seen.

It is important to advise premenopausal women that adequate contraception is essential while undergoing a course of cheotherapy. Generally, medical advice should be sought as to when it is safe to conceive after a course of chemotherapy has finished.

SELF-IMAGE

It is important for nurses to pay attention to the effects cytotoxic therapy can have on patients' self-image. Many of those undergoing chemotherapy will have already experienced the changes to self-image that surgery can cause and some will have been deeply affected. Now the patient is facing treatment that may reduce her physical and mental capabilities and cause her to be unable to function normally in her various roles, e.g. as wife, mother, worker, etc. This may also have implications for the financial security of her and her family.

Furthermore, chemotherapy often has an effect on the patient's sexuality, and can cause loss of libido, dry vagina and other physical and psychological sexual problems (Chapter 15). Counselling by the nurse may be helpful, but some patients will need referral to a specialist sexual counsellor.

MEASURING RESPONSE

It is vital that patients are monitored regularly to assess their response to the chemotherapy as well as checking for toxicity. It is quite usual for patients to receive more than one regime of chemotherapy over time. The objective gauging of response includes measuring any visible tumour and metastases visible on scan or X-ray.

These must not be taken as the only measurement, however. The patient must be assessed as a whole, and the quality of her life must be fully taken into account when deciding on further treatment. Furthermore, and very importantly, the patient must be fully involved in any decisions taken about treatment. In this context the role of the nurse is to be an advocate, ensuring the patient has all the necessary information to be able to participate in the decision-making, and then supporting her in the decision she takes.

FOR THE FUTURE

Some research has been carried out examining the role of tumour markers in the blood and urine in order to identify substances whose levels would indicate response or progression of the disease. Although this research is in its early stages it offers hope that changes in blood results could lead to earlier more responsive treatment, thus improving the quality of life for patients with advanced breast cancer. There have also been studies looking at the use of chemotherapy given into the mammary artery; this could be an important tool in future breast cancer management.

CONCLUSION

Chemotherapy can be used to treat women suffering from all stages of breast cancer. While chemotherapy is not without side-effects, some of them quite distressing, these effects are being reduced as the drugs and regimes are refined and improved. Good medical and nursing care is vital for all patients, especially those suffering side-effects. Finally, it is vital that all members of the breast care team work well together so as to minimize the side-effects of cytotoxic chemotherapy and optimize it as a method of treatment for patients with breast cancer.

REFERENCES

Speechley, V. in Tiffany, R. and Borely, D. (1989). *Oncology for Nurses and Health Care Professionals*, Volume 3, Harper and Row.

Bonadonna, G. *et al.* (1985), Ten year experience with CMF based adjuvent chemotherapy in resectable breast cancer. *Breast Cancer Res. and Treatment*, **5**, 95–115.

Ahmann, D.L. *et al.* (1984) Status of adjuvent chemotherapy in patients with breast cancer. *Cancer* (Supplement), **53**, 724–8.

Spittle, M.F. *et al.* (1986) Adjuvent chemotherapy in the treatment of breast cancer: results of a multi-centre study. *Euro. Jnl Surg. Oncol.*, **12**, 109–16.

Early Breast Cancer Trialists Collaterative Group (1990) *Treatment of Early Breast Cancer*, Volume 1 Worldwide Evidence 1985–1990, Oxford University Press, Oxford.

Endocrine therapies for breast cancer

8

Deborah Fenlon

INTRODUCTION

Endocrine therapy is the most elegant form of treatment for breast cancer as it uses the body's own mechanisms to fight the cancer and is less invasive or toxic than other methods. The 'mechanisms' behind this treatment give an insight into the nature of breast cancer, and so may lead to better understanding of the causes of the disease and thus the possibility of preventing it.

Unfortunately, endocrine therapy is currently only useful in some women and can at best lead to slowing the progress of the disease, not cure. It is important to remember this when assessing the efficacy of treatment for patients receiving endocrine therapy as their quality of life must be the paramount consideration when cure is not a possibility.

HISTORICAL PERSPECTIVE

It has been known for many years that hormonal treatment is effective in certain types of cancer. In 1896, Beatson noticed that oophorectomy obtained a response in women with advanced breast cancer (Beatson, 1896). Later it was found that adrenalectomy and hypophysectomy were also useful for hormone-dependent tumours (Huggins and Bergenstal, 1952).

However, these treatments also caused a high degree of morbidity and mortality, so chemical methods were sought that would have the same effectiveness but be reversible, allowing treatment to be stopped if necessary.

In the 1960's the anticonvulsant drug aminoglutethimide was found to cause adrenal inhibition and subsequently came to be useful in treating breast cancer. Since then many more drugs have proved to be useful, including androgens, progesterones and more selective inhibitors of oestrogen production. Others, offering improved efficacy and minimal toxicity, are constantly being developed.

The most successful drug to date is an antioestrogen called tamoxifen, which was originally investigated as a fertility drug (Jordan, 1986). This is generally now the first choice of endocrine treatment in advanced cancer. It is also being used in conjunction with surgery for primary breast cancer as it can delay the onset of recurrence; and the possibility of its having a role in the prevention of breast cancer is even being investigated.

The use of hormone treatments in breast cancer has contributed greatly to an understanding of the disease process itself. A significant step was made in 1959 when hormone receptor sites were first demonstrated. This was shown when radioactively-labelled oestrogens were selectively taken up by hormone-dependent organs in the body. Patients who had a high uptake of the radiolabel were also the ones who responded better to adrenalectomy (Casey, 1981). It was therefore proposed that oestrogen receptor (ER) sites exist in hormone-responsive tissue. Progesterone sites have now also been demonstrated.

It is hoped that studies of hormones will ultimately show what causes breast cancer and how to cure or even prevent it.

PHYSIOLOGY

Hormone production

Hormones are substances produced by glands in one part of the body that exert an influence elsewhere in the body. The hormones that are useful in the treatment of breast cancer are the sex hormones. These are mainly produced in the gonads (ovaries and testes), which are under the control of the pituitary gland and the hypothalamus (Figure 8.1). The hypothalamus produces luteinizing hormone-releasing hormone (LHRH) which stimulates the pituitary to release more complex hormone such as luteinizing hormone (LH), follicle-stimulating hormone (FSH) and adrenocorticotrophic hormone (ACTH). These in turn stimulate the adrenal gland to produce corticosteroids, and the ovaries to produce oestrogens.

Steroid hormone receptors

Most hormones are carried in the blood by plasma proteins such as sex hormone binding globulin (SHBG) When the hormone reaches the cell it enters by diffusion. In order to enter the nucleus and exert an influence the hormone

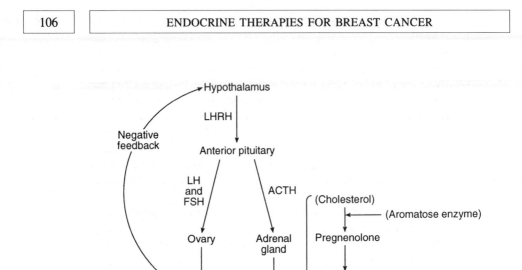

Figure 8.1 Pathways of oestrogen and progesterone production.

must bind to a receptor protein found in the cell cytoplasm. Once bound to the receptor protein, the hormone crosses to the nucleus where it stimulates growth. Oestrogen receptors (ER) are measured in femtomoles per milligram of cytoplasmic protein, ranging from 0 to more than 1000. If the concentration of ER is above 10 Fmol/mg then it is said to be ER-positive (Osborne, 1985).

Negative feedback control

Control of the above processes is by a negative feedback system. When the level of end-product hormones such as oestrogen is high, the hypothalamus and pituitary gland are inhibited from producing stimulating hormones.

Steroid hormones

All steroid hormones are related to cholesterol. The adrenal gland synthesizes and secretes all the steroid hormones – glucocorticoids, mineralocorticoids, androgens, oestrogens and progesterones. The most important of these is hydrocortisone, which affects all the tissues in the body and is essential to life. Cortisone, prednisolone and dexamethasone are all drugs that behave like hydrocortisone. The amount of sex hormones produced in the adrenals is relatively small but becomes more significant in the post-menopausal woman.

The testes and the ovaries produce both androgens and oestrogens, but in different amounts. Androgens are responsible for the development of male genitalia and other virilizing effects. They also have an anabolic effect, causing the development of muscle and skeletal tissue. Oestrogens and progesterones are responsible for the development of the breasts, and are also important in the regulation of menstruation, lactation and pregnancy.

Tumour behaviour

Cancers that arise in hormone-dependent organs appear to need appropriate hormones for their growth. Depriving breast cancer of oestrogen has been shown to cause tumour regression.

ER-positive tumours seem to be better differentiated, i.e. they are more like the original tissue, and less aggressive than ER-negative ones. They are more common in post-menopausal women and are associated with better prognosis, a longer disease-free interval and longer survival.

Between 50% and 60% of breast cancers are ER-positive and of these 60% will respond to hormone therapies; overall the response rate is 30% (Powles, 1983). Those that are ER-negative are unlikely to respond to hormone treatment, and Goodman (1988) suggests that this knowledge spares those with hormone insensitive tumours from 'the wasted effort of hormone therapy'. However, about 10% of ER-negative tumours do respond to hormone therapy so there are occasions when it may be useful.

Hormone therapy does not kill all the cancer cells, and does not therefore cure the patient; this is because a cancer comprises a mix of cell populations in which some of the cells are hormone-sensitive and others are not. Therefore, when a hormone treatment is given all the sensitive cells in the population are killed leaving the insensitive cells to grow and cause the cancer to recur. Also, if one source of oestrogen is wiped out, other sources will eventually take over and cause the cancer cells to grow. However, if the cancer becomes resistant to one hormone treatment another may still cause a response by cutting a different source of oestrogen or by hitting a different cell population.

Clinical use

In summary, hormone treatment is more likely to be useful in post-menopausal women, particularly those with high ER receptivity. It is also important to note that these treatments are likely to take six to eight weeks before having a noticeable effect; they are therefore not useful when the patient has rapidly-progressing or life-threatening disease.

CLINICAL USES OF HORMONAL MANIPULATION

Preventive

The possibility of using tamoxifen to prevent breast cancer is currently a controversial issue. There is much evidence to show it could be successful, but many people argue that there is as yet insufficient evidence about long-term side-effects.

It is thought that oestrogens are involved in the causation of breast cancer; tamoxifen is an antioestrogen and it therefore seems likely that it could protect the breast from the stimulation of oestrogen. It is also known that tamoxifen protects mice exposed to a carcinogenic agent from developing breast cancer (Jordan, 1986). Patients who have had breast cancer in one breast and are then treated with adjuvant tamoxifen appear to have a reduced risk of developing cancer in the other breast (Early Breast Cancer Trialists Collaborative Group, 1992).

Worries about the use of tamoxifen in a population of healthy women centre on the unknown. It has been suggested that there may be adverse effects on the reproductive tract and blood clotting factors (leading to possible thrombo-embolic disorders), an increased risk of osteoporosis, and possible retinal damage. There is currently little evidence to support these worries. Indeed, some figures have shown that women receiving tamoxifen as an adjuvant therapy have a lower risk of dying of heart-related problems than the normal population (Stewart, 1992). It has recently been found that tamoxifen treatment is associated with a modest increase in endometrial carcinoma (Jordan and Morrow, 1994).

Adjuvant therapy

Hormone treatment, begun at the time of the initial diagnosis of breast cancer and given alongside primary surgery, can prolong the disease-free interval and may increase overall survival. Tamoxifen is the most commonly used drug in this connection, although the effect has also been demonstrated with other hormones such as aminoglutethimide. This effect is only seen in post-menopausal women, most strongly in those with oestrogen receptor-positive tumours.

Metastatic therapy

The use of hormonal agents in advanced breast cancer is of great value. Once breast cancer has recurred it is not generally thought to be curable. It is therefore paramount that the patient does not deem the treatments to be worse than the disease as quality, rather than quantity, of life becomes more relevant at this stage. Hormone therapies have a great role to play in this area as they can be very effective and yet are associated with relatively low toxicity.

Oophorectomy and LHRH agonists

As discussed above, the presence of oestrogens appears to stimulate the growth of breast cancer; the rationale of treatment is therefore to decrease or oppose the action of oestrogens. In pre-menopausal women this is achieved by oophorectomy, either by radiotherapy or surgery. The use of drugs, such as Zoladex, buserelin and leuprorelin, is now also an option.

The hypothalamus secretes LHRH which stimulates the pituitary to release gonadotrophic hormones, inducing secretion of oestrogens from the ovary. Analogues of LHRH are about 100 times more potent than LHRH itself. If given in low doses they could stimulate the pituitary, but if given in large doses they desensitize receptors on the pituitary cell surface, inhibiting the release of gonadotrophins and leading to a castration-like effect (Furr and Milsted, 1988).

These drugs are just as effective as oophorectomy, but have less morbidity and their effect is reversible. The most convenient formulation is Zoladex, as it can be given by a subcutaneous depot injection once a month. Others are given subcutaneously, intranasally or by vaginal pessaries. They will all cause some menopausal symptoms, but otherwise side-effects are rare.

Adjuvant chemotherapy has been shown to obtain a survival benefit for pre-menopausal women. It may be that this effect is brought about by the suppression of the ovaries; Padmanabhan, Howell and Rubens (1986) reported that the therapeutic effects of adjuvant chemotherapy were only found in women in whom permanent amenorrhoea had been induced. If this is the case, giving an LHRH analogue would be just as effective as, and far more easily tolerated than, chemotherapy.

Adrenal ablation and aromatase inhibitors

The ovaries are the main source of oestrogens but post-menopausal women still produce some oestrogen. The adrenal glands produce precursors such as androstenedione which is converted to oestrogen by the action of the enzyme aromatase. This process occurs in extraglandular tissue such as fat and is not under negative feedback control.

In the past this process was prevented by adrenalectomy or hypophysectomy, and significant regression of the cancer was seen. However, since the introduction of aminoglutethimide these operations are no longer carried out. Aminoglutethimide is an inhibitor of all adrenal hormone synthesis and of the non-adrenal conversion of androgens to oestrogens. It is therefore a very effective drug in the treatment of breast cancer, but it also has a high incidence of side-effects. Acute toxicity may be present in up to 50% of patients (Cavalli, 1989). Symptoms suffered are severe drowsiness, ataxia or rash. Nausea or diarrhoea may also occur, and blood disorders are rare complications. The rash is usually mild and will resolve, but it can be very severe and accompanied by a fever. In extreme cases exfoliation can occur. Tolerance to the side-effects may develop, but 10% of patients may need to discontinue use of the drug, mainly because of chronic toxicity, such as depression.

Because aminoglutethimide also inhibits hydrocortisone production, the subsequent negative feedback stimulation of the pituitary may lead to increased stimulation of the adrenals to produce more hormones and overcome the beneficial effect of the aminoglutethimide. For this reason hydrocortisone replacement is given. If therapy is discontinued the hydrocortisone must be gradually reduced in order to allow the adrenals time to recover their function or adrenal insufficiency may occur and the patient suffer an Addisonian crisis.

In view of these problems, many new drugs are under investigation to replace aminoglutethimide. One of these is formestane (Leutaron). This is an aromatase inhibitor which does not inhibit the adrenal gland but does inhibit the conversion of androstenedione to oestrogen. It can be given orally in daily doses of 500mg or as a fortnightly intramuscular injection. There have been very few side-effects noted with this drug. Sterile abscesses can form at the site of administration of the injection.

Oestrogen therapy

Large doses of oestrogen, such as diethylstilboestrol, are therapeutic in post-menopausal women. This is apparently because large doses of oestrogen will constantly occupy the oestrogen receptor site and interfere with the stimulatory process. However, oestrogens often cause a 'flare' in which the disease is initially stimulated before seeing a regression. This is manifested by an increase in local disease or bone pain, and hypercalcaemia may occur. Oestrogens also have severe side-effects, such as fluid retention, which could exacerbate cardiac failure in the elderly, and can also cause thrombo-embolic and cardiovascular problems. They are therefore rarely used now.

Androgen therapy

The administration of androgens, such as Durabolin, nandrolone, fluoxy-mesterone or testosterone will result in tumour regression in 60–70% of women who have oestrogen and androgen receptors present in their tumour (Goodman, 1988). It is uncertain how they work. It may be due to the androgens binding to the oestrogen receptor or by their exerting a negative feedback effect to the pituitary, therefore inhibiting production of oestrogens.

However, these too produce severe side-effects and so are now rarely used. Side-effects used are those of masculinization, such as hirsuitism, deepening of the voice and male pattern hair loss. The skin may also thicken and become coarser and increased oil production can lead to acne. An initial feeling of euphoria and general well-being may be induced, but this will soon wear off.

Progestin therapy

Progesterone seems to be the natural antagonist of oestrogen. In breast cancer it appears to work by opposing the natural stimulating action of oestrogen. It may do this by acting via the progesterone receptor to reduce the number of oestrogen receptors. Progestogens used are medroxyprogesterone acetate, megestrol acetate and norethisterone. They are associated with a much lower incidence of side-effects than androgens. The most frequent problem is weight gain and increased appetite. Hot flushes are not seen but occasionally there is increased perspiration and night sweats. Latent diabetes may become overt. Cushingoid features such as a 'moon face' can occur with medroxyprogesterone acetate. As with the androgens, a significant percentage of patients experience a sense of well-being.

Progestins may be useful if given in conjunction with chemotherapy as they appear to reduce myelosuppression and will combat weight loss.

Tamoxifen

Tamoxifen is an antioestrogen. It competes with oestrogen to bind to the oestrogen receptor site, but once there does not cause growth stimulation as oestrogen would do. In other ways it may act as a mild oestrogen. The main side-effects are hot flushes and vaginal discharge and it is generally the drug of first choice in the treatment of breast cancer. 'Flare' is seen with the use of tamoxifen in up to 2% of patients (Vallis and Waxman, 1988).

Corticosteroids

Corticosteroids such as prednisolone are known to have an anticancer effect, but it is shortlived and they are therefore not particularly useful as a treatment option. They do appear to enhance the effect of chemotherapy, and so may be given as part of a chemotherapeutic regime. They can also be useful for controlling symptoms such as bone pain, shortness of breath and irritation from skin metastases. Dexamethasone is used to relieve the symptoms of cerebral and spinal mestastases by reduction of local oedema.

In terminal patients, steroids may also boost the appetite and give a short but welcome lift to their morale by providing a feeling of well-being. Short courses of steroids may also be given to try to prevent the sickness associated with chemotherapy, but this needs to be carefully monitored as some patients suffer a withdrawal effect when stopping the steroid and this may be worse than the problem it was given to counter.

Summary of clinical use

In advanced cancer hormone therapy is used for patients who have non-life-threatening disease, usually of the skin or bones. When the cancer is aggressive or affects lung or liver, chemotherapy must be used as hormone therapy may be too slow to be effective.

In pre-menopausal women the main aim is to prevent the ovaries from working. This is achieved either by oophorectomy or the use of Zoladex. In post-menopausal women there are many choices of action. Treatment now nearly always involves the use of drugs rather than surgery. The best currently available drug is tamoxifen. The new aromatase inhibitors will probably become the second treatment of choice due to their low incidence of side-effects, holding the progestins in reserve. The androgens, oestrogens and aminoglutethimide will probably now become rare.

The response rate for all the hormone treatments is similar, being about 30% overall and 60–70% for ER-positive patients. The mean duration of response is about 20 months. There appears to be little advantage in combining different endocrine therapies but there may be a role for giving endocrine therapy alongside chemotherapy.

Treatment of male breast cancer

Carcinoma of the male breast constitutes only 1% of all breast cancer. Primary treatment is by surgery and radiotherapy, as for women. Hormone treatment has been based on experience with women, which is not necessarily transferable. However, the collection of relevant data is difficult as there are so few subjects available; therefore no consensus has been reached about the best method of treatment for this group.

Oestrogen receptors are present in 89% of male breast cancers, and 71% are positive for progesterone receptors (Crichlow and Evans, 1987). This would appear to indicate that this group is particularly suitable for hormone manipulation. Orchidectomy is generally the first line treatment, with a response rate of about 55%. However, this is not always acceptable to the patient and the use of tamoxifen, with a response of 46%, may be preferable. Aminoglutethimide and the progesterones have also been shown to be of benefit.

PROBLEMS FACED BY PATIENTS ON HORMONE THERAPY, AND NURSING INTERVENTIONS

Quality of life

Patients receiving hormonal therapy are often those whose disease has already spread and for whom the treatment is not a cure. Dunne (1988) suggests that the goal of care may be mobility, absence of pain and the ability to function at work or at home. This is a significant factor in choosing treatment options and in assessing the degree of side-effects suffered by a patient. If the perceived side-effects are very great the patient may choose to forgo that particular treatment option. However, side-effects are generally low and hormone therapy is thus regarded as an effective way of increasing length and quality of life. Nursing interventions to help overcome any problems the patient is suffering may be important in improving the patient's acceptance of the drugs.

The majority of patients in this group are women between the ages of 40 and 65. They often have vital family roles as wives and mothers and their relationships within the family must be taken into account when assessing the problems the patient may be facing.

It is also important to remember that although many of these patients have potentially terminal cancer, they often remain well enough to be treated as out-patients for much of their illness. Most of the nurses they meet will therefore be out-patient nurses, who thus have a duty to be well informed and prepared to get to know the patients. Sque (1985) has stressed the importance of out-patient nurses forming these relationships and of providing continuity of care. She also says that if patients have allies in their battles it will help them trade their fears for confidence.

Menopausal symptoms

Menopausal symptoms are suffered by many women being treated for breast cancer. The menopause may be induced as part of the treatment; for example, adjuvant chemotherapy may stop menstruation. Women who are receiving hormone replacement therapy (HRT) will suffer a return of their symptoms when this treatment is discontinued; HRT is usually not advisable when a woman has breast cancer. Many other hormone treatments also have some menopausal symptoms as side-effects. A large part of this chapter is therefore devoted to menopausal symptoms, even though not all patients are actually going through the menopause.

To help patients cope with these experiences the nurse's first task is information-giving and education. Initially this will tend to be in terms of explaining the treatment programme and the onset of symptoms in relation to the treatment. For example, where ovarian function is suppressed gradually, as with adjuvant chemotherapy, the nurse must explain why it is necessary to continue to use an effective and safe method of birth control. The patient must fully understand the complications that may arise for both the mother and the foetus if an unplanned pregnancy occurs. Knowledge must be reassessed and information reinforced as part of an ongoing educational process.

Some women will pass through the menopause without suffering any problems at all while others may have severe symptoms lasting for years. A great variety of symptoms have been described but the most common is the hot flush, experienced by 55% of women. Other common symptoms are: tiredness (40%), nervousness (41%), abnormal sweating (39%), headaches (38%), insomnia (32%) and depression (30%) (Howie, 1987). It is not known whether an artificially-induced menopause is prone to the same degree of symptoms as a natural one, although hot flushes do not appear to be influenced (Levine-Silverman, 1989).

General measures to help menopausal symptoms

As well as the more obvious symptoms discussed below, there are many non-specific symptoms associated with menopause that can be very difficult to alleviate by direct methods. These include physical symptoms such as:

- backache
- constipation
- decreased sex drive
- palpitations
- giddiness
- water retention
- generalized aches and pains.

There are also many mental symptoms including:

- anxiety
- loss of concentration
- panic attacks
- confusion
- loss of confidence
- irritability.

It is important that the nurse first recognizes the source of these problems and is able to help the patient understand what is happening to her. Very often the woman is frightened about the changes occurring and does not realize that they are due to the menopause; 25% of women do not even discuss their menopause with anyone (Voda, 1986).

A number of theories are currently being presented about the role of diet in helping menopausal symptoms, but there is as yet little evidence to support them. The Women's Nutritional Advisory Service (WNAS) provides a nutritional and lifestyle programme which it claims to have helped women reduce their menopausal symptoms. Most of the WNAS' advice on diet follows the generally accepted line of reducing fat, sugar and salt and increasing consumption of fresh fruit, vegetables and cereals. It also recommends taking supplements of magnesium, calcium and other trace elements along with various vitamins. Vitamin B6 is thought to be useful for mental disturbance problems and insomnia, and vitamin E is recommended to help control hot flushes (Howie, 1987). Some groups also believe oil of evening primrose to be of benefit.

It is thought that women who exercise regularly have fewer menopausal symptoms than those who do not. A package of regular exercise and relaxation may also help to decrease menopausal problems.

Specific measures to help menopausal symptoms

Flushes and sweats

Hot flushes are the most common problem at the menopause. It is unclear what triggers them or why they occur. They can be short, mild and infrequent, but they have been reported at a frequency of up to 240 in a 24-hour period and 14% women describe them as severe (Levine-Silverman, 1989). Many women also describe increased sweating and night sweats as being a problem.

Various hormonal methods have been tried to alleviate hot flushing. Oestrogen replacement therapy is the most effective, but would normally be contra-indicated in patients with breast cancer. Progesterone therapy may also be effective. Clonidine and ethamsylate have been shown to be of some use in controlling sweats. These are not hormones but have a local vasoconstricting effect.

Some people find that flushes are triggered by hot drinks, alcohol or hot spicy foods. It may be worth suggesting the patient try avoiding these for a time to see if flushing can be reduced. Smoking may also be implicated, so this should be cut down.

Comfort may be increased by wearing thin layers of clothing that can easily be peeled off if a flush occurs and by using lightweight layers of bed clothing at night. Cotton is more absorbent and so remains comfortable even after a sweat. Carrying moist tissues or a hand-held electric fan can help cooling and be refreshing. Unaccustomed exercise and stress will aggravate flushing and so should be avoided. It may be possible for the patient to learn biofeedback control to decrease the intensity of flushes.

Physical means may help reduce the discomfort of flushing but do not normally prevent it from occurring; learning coping strategies may therefore be more important. Facing the flushes with a positive attitude – even humour may not decrease the discomfort but may make the experience less distressing. Distraction or trying to concentrate on something else may reduce the impact of the flush, although women often report that flushes distract them from what they were doing, so concentration is obviously diminished.

The flush is usually perceived as being a much greater event by the sufferer than by the people around her, so embarrassment is also a problem. If the woman can be reassured that the flush is not nearly as obvious to others as she believes the embarrassment can be reduced.

Osteoporosis

It is known that once oestrogen levels are reduced in the body the bones have a tendency to lose calcium and become brittle. This process of osteoporosis is not fully understood and at present it is impossible to prevent it. The only factors known to reduce osteoporosis in old age are an adequate intake of calcium in the pre-pubertal girl and the participation in regular weight-bearing exercise throughout life. Taking calcium supplements as an adult has been shown to be ineffective.

Other factors, such as an increase in magnesium intake and a decrease in smoking have been suggested, but none are proven.

Skin and hair

Once past menopause, oily secretions dry up and the skin and hair start to become dry and age more rapidly. Many women, especially those going through an early artificial menopause, worry that they will quickly begin to look old. This ageing process cannot be reversed, but it is worth reassuring the woman that the effects will not be immediately noticeable and that the onset of ageing will be gradual and slow.

It is worthwhile keeping the skin in good condition by using richer moisturizing lotions and make-up. Using milder soaps and avoiding detergents will help the skin preserve what natural oils are left. Less frequent washing of the hair and the use of richer hair conditioners will help keep the hair in good condition. There is much discussion about the role of vitamin E and evening primrose oil in slowing down ageing and many people take supplements for this purpose. Certainly, an adequate intake of the vitamin B group is important for the health of skin, hair and nails, but this can be achieved by a good balanced diet.

Vaginal atrophy (dryness, irritation and dyspareunia)

The decrease in production of natural oils also affects the vagina. This means that less lubrication is produced during intercourse leading to difficult, and possibly painful, sex. The skin around the vagina will also become dryer and lose its elasticity, which may also lead to problems with sexual intercourse. Vaginal atrophy may be associated with considerable irritation and soreness.

In general, it is recommended that sexual intercourse should be continued to aid circulation and maintain tissue elasticity. Lubrication may be provided by use of a pharmaceutical gel such as K-Y Jelly. If the atrophy causes the vagina to become very narrow the use of a dilator may become necessary. If vaginal irritation is a problem oestrogen cream is contra-indicated because of the high level of absorption into the blood stream that occurs in this area. Hydrocortisone cream may be used, but only under medical supervision as this is also absorbed into the blood stream. A soothing cream may help and treatment must be aimed at preventing infection by careful cleansing with mild soaps and gentle but thorough drying. Thrush is an opportunistic infective agent that can be troublesome in this situation so antifungal cream may be used.

Depression

It is uncertain whether menopausal depression is due to the biological changes taking place within the woman or whether it is largely the result of concurrent changes in lifestyle. For many the menopause frequently coincides with the time in their life when her role is undergoing major shift as her children leave home. The end of her reproductive function may make a woman aware that she is getting older. This may make her feel less attractive sexually and that she is less desirable as a sexual partner. Many women also realize that without the protection of oestrogens the body will age more rapidly, so the menopause can mark the beginning of a woman feeling 'old'.

It is interesting to note that in societies where women gain status at menopause there are fewer reports of menopausal symptoms (Voda, 1986). Voda's study looked at Rajput women who were able to sit with men and participate in decision-making in village management only after ceasing to menstruate.

Problems with loss of role as a mother and wife, loss of self-esteem as a result of ageing and a decrease in feelings of being attractive are all enhanced in the cancer patient since the disease itself can also cause body image problems and interfere with everyday functioning. A woman on hormone therapy is also usually suffering from recurrent cancer and may therefore be facing real fears about her own mortality. It may consequently be considered normal for a woman to show some signs of depression at this time, but it is important that the nurse adequately assesses the degree of depression and refers the woman for medical or psychiatric help where appropriate.

Body image and sexuality

The problems a patient with breast cancer may have with her body image as a result of surgery are well known, but those caused by hormonal treatments are not so widely discussed. They are many and varied, ranging from mild weight gain through the Cushingoid 'moon face' to virilization, such as facial hair growth and irreversible voice changes. As hormone treatments are usually given after surgery, the woman has already suffered one blow to her body integrity. She may also now be suffering advanced disease which may itself be causing some problems with self-image. Patients on hormonal therapies may therefore be experiencing threats to their body image from a multiplicity of sources.

Feldman (1989) suggests that body image, sexuality and self-esteem are all closely linked and that poor self-esteem can lead to a negative body image and problems with sexuality. Webb (1985) defines self-esteem as the product of a positive self-concept and clear body image linked to feelings of autonomy, independence and the ability to make decisions.

These definitions can help us work out programmes to help women in this situation. Autonomy can be increased by helping women take control of their disease and treatment. This is best done by giving full and clear information and guiding women to make treatment choices based on their own priorities and goals. Nurses can help define goals, emphasize positive experiences and identify new coping strategies.

An increase in self-esteem will help overcome problems with body image, but some direct measures can be taken as well. For example, some women may have an unrealistic image of themselves and the nurse can help them to rationalize these feelings. Many patients perceive their hot flushes to be obvious to everyone around them when this is frequently not so.

These problems with changed body image, coupled with physical problems and the emotional disturbances that a patient on hormone therapy may have, can lead to sexual difficulties. The nurse needs to establish a rapport with the patient to give her a safe environment in which to discuss these problems if she wishes to. The nurse must be non-judgemental, non-threatening and reassuring.

In discussing changes in practice, such as the use of lubricants, it is useful to concentrate on how the patient feels rather than on the technicalities. Some patients feel they need to conserve their energies for coping with their illness so that sex becomes less important, and many partners also feel this way. It is therefore necessary to establish what is important for both partners and to help them to work out common goals. Other forms of expressing love and affection may become more important to the couple while they find that 'normal' sexual intercourse becomes a lower priority. Most couples are able to adjust to these changes in their relationship but some may find referral to a sexual counsellor helpful.

Menstrual disturbances

Drugs that induce the menopause will obviously cause menstruation to cease, but other hormones may cause menstrual changes as well. Tamoxifen can cause periods to become lighter in pre-menopausal women; more rarely it may cause periods to be heavier. Post-menopausal women sometimes have a withdrawal bleed when oestrogens or tamoxifen are discontinued. This can be very alarming if it is unexpected, so patients should be warned of the possibility. The woman should always be encouraged to seek medical advice if she experiences any abnormal vaginal discharge or bleeding.

Gastrointestinal disturbances

Some hormonal therapies, such as tamoxifen, cause mild, transient nausea needing little intervention other than explanation and reassurance that it will soon pass. Others, such as the oestrogens, may cause more severe nausea and possibly vomiting, which will require treatment with anti-emetics. It is important to observe the course of the nausea in case it is a symptom of 'flare' and is caused by hypercalcaemia. Diarrhoea is a rare complication but may be caused by aminoglutethimide. If it does not pass quickly treatment may need to be interrupted.

Weight change

The progestins, especially medroxyprogesterone acetate, can cause an increase in appetite and may well result in weight gain. Some women find this particularly distressing if they are already suffering feelings of poor self-image because of other factors in their cancer treatment. But weight gain is not inevitable and women can attempt to keep their weight down with a careful diet. Tamoxifen can also cause an increase in weight. It is generally a small gain, but it is important to warn women that it is a side-effect so they are forewarned and able to take steps to control it if they wish.

Sexual problems

A change in the libido can be a direct effect of hormone therapy as well as an indirect one: oestrogens, for example, can reduce the libido. This may not be a problem for some women but many breast cancer patients have active sexual relationships. These effects must be considered alongside the other possible difficulties in sexual relationships discussed above, and the patient should be given appropriate support and counselling. Oestrogen treatment is not often given any more.

Progesterones and androgens can increase the libido. Again, this may not necessarily be a problem for the individual, indeed it could be a beneficial effect of the treatment; however, as it could present a problem for some, the effect should not be ignored.

Virilization

Some hormones, particularly androgens, will cause masculinizing changes. These can be very distressing for the patient, especially if she is not warned about them. Some of the changes, such as deepening of the voice, may not be reversible. Earlier changes are an increased secretion of sebum causing oily skin and acne. The skin itself may thicken and become coarser. Male pattern hair loss may be seen and facial hirsuitism can occcur.

These changes cannot be prevented so it is largely a matter of helping the patient to adjust to them. Acne and oily skin can be kept to a minimum by taking a good diet with plenty of fresh fruit and vegetables and reducing fat intake. Facial hair is best dealt with by bleaching or electrolysis as shaving will cause the hair to thicken and result in blue shadowing on the face.

Drug reactions

The most common reaction to hormonal treatment is the aminoglutethimide rash. This is very frequent and can be very severe. If it is mild the patient is asked to continue the drug as the effect will wear off. A soothing lotion such as calamine will help ease the discomfort and Piriton taken at night may help reduce the itching and give a good night's sleep. The rash may be accompanied by fever, lethargy and a general feeling of being very unwell, in which case the doctor must be informed and the drug may need to be discontinued. The patient must know about these effects so that she can report them if they occur.

Particular problems for men

Breast cancer is a rare disease in men and they have a unique set of problems. First, because it is rare and because it is a 'female' disease they are likely to feel very isolated. In the absence of fellow sufferers for them to talk to about the illness, medical staff should make particular time to provide this kind of support.

The hormonal treatments will all have a feminizing effect, such as gynaecomastia, and the consequent feelings of having been demasculinized may exacerbate the patient's sense of isolation. The hormones are also likely to cause loss of libido, even impotence, so a man is going to suffer sexual problems as well. The same kind of interventions used for women are effective.

Steroid effects

Steroids are not usually used for very long periods in treatment programmes for breast cancer, so many of the long-term side-effects are not seen. Nevertheless, some of the early changes are seen and the side-effects can be severe and so should be known about. The collective symptoms are known as Cushing's syndrome and include:

- development of fat 'moon face'
- redistribution of body fat to give truncal obesity, fat hump on shoulders and wasted limbs;
- acne;
- thinning of hair on head;
- facial hirsuitism;
- muscle weakness;
- striae and ease of bruising;
- osteoporosis;
- diabetes mellitus.

The physical changes are seen when high doses of steroids are given for cranial irradiation, and they can be very distressing to the patient. The benefit of the treatment must be carefully explained to make the side-effects tolerable. Other ways of coping are careful diet (although this will not prevent moon face) and advice on make-up and beauty care. As discussed previously, it may help the patient to be able to talk through her feelings about her body image and self-esteem.

When steroids are given over a long period of time the body's ability to make hydrocortisone is impaired. This means the body would not be able to cope with stressful situations if the steroid were suddenly discontinued. The patient and her family must therefore understand that if she is unable to take her medication for any reason she should inform her doctor or she may become seriously ill. Any patient taking steroid drugs should carry a card at all times giving details of the drug in case of emergency.

Because of the possibility of developing diabetes the patient should also have her urine tested at regular intervals.

Cardiovascular problems

The use of oestrogens is associated with cardiovascular problems. They can cause an increased risk of thrombo-embolism and therefore pose a danger to the patient. For this reason they are now rarely used, but it is necessary for the nurses to know of the risks and observe for them when these drugs are still used. They can also cause fluid retention, which may exacerbate congestive cardiac failure in the elderly.

Flare

The term 'flare' is used to describe a rare situation that can occur with hormonal therapy of an initial worsening of the cancer before a response takes place. This is manifested by an increase in bone pain and possible reaction in skin nodules. It is important to note because hypercalcaemia can occur and this may be life-threatening. The usual symptoms of hypercalcaemia should be looked for, i.e. thirst, confusion, nausea and constipation. It is most commonly seen in patients taking oestrogens and may also occur in those taking tamoxifen.

SUMMARY

From the above discussion it would appear that there are many problems associated with the use of hormone therapies. These have been emphasized so that nurses can be aware of them and help patients to face and overcome them. However, the modern hormonal drugs that are now available offer considerable relief to many women with breast cancer while causing relatively little in the way of side-effects. So long as medical staff are able to support breast cancer patients and help them to have autonomy over their illness and treatment, hormone therapies are of great benefit.

REFERENCES

Beatson, G.T. (1896) On the management of inoperable cases of carcinoma of the mamma: suggestion for new method of treatment with illustrative cases. *Lancet*, 2, 104–7, 162–5.

Casey, A. (1981) Oestrogen receptor and breast cancer. *Nursing Times*, 16 April.

Cavalli, F. (1989) *Endocrine Therapy of Breast Cancer III*, Springer-Verlag, Berlin.

Crichlow, R.W. and Evans, D.B. (1987) Cancer in the Male Breast, in *Breast Cancer: Diagnosis and Treatment* (ed. I. Ariel and J. Cleary), McGraw-Hill, New York.

Dunne, C.F. (1988) Hormonal therapy for breast cancer. *Cancer Nursing* 11(5), 288–94.

Early Breast Cancer Trialist's Collaborative Group (1992) Systemic treatment of early breast cancer by hormonal, cytotoxic or immune therapy. *The Lancet*, 339(8784), 1–15.

Feldman, J.E. (1989) Ovarian failure and cancer treatment: incidence and interventions for the premenopausal woman. *Oncology Nursing Forum*, 16(5), 651–7.

Furr, B.J.A. and Milsted, R.A.V. (1988) LH–RH Analogues in Cancer Treatment in *Endocrine Management of Cancer: Volume 2 Contemporary Therapy* (ed. B. Stoll), Karger, Basle.

Goodman, M. (1988) Concepts of hormonal manipulation in the treatment of cancer. *Oncology Nursing Forum*, 15(5), 639–47.

Howie, C. (1987) Sparing the flushes. *Nursing Times*, 83(49), 51–3.

Huggins, C. and Bergenstal, D.M. (1952) Inhibition of human mammary and prostatic cancer by adrenalectomy. *Cancer Research*, 12, 134–41.

Jordan, V.C. (1986) *Estrogen/Antiestrogen Action and Breast Cancer Therapy*, Wisconsin Press, Madison.

Jordan, V.C. and Morrow, M. (1994) Should clinicians be concerned about the carcinogenic potential of tamoxifen? *European Journal of Cancer*, 30A(11), 1714–21.

Levine-Silverman, S. (1989) The menopausal hot flash: a procrustean bed of research. *Journal of Advanced Nursing*, **14**, 939–49.

Osborne, C.K. (1985) Heterogeneity in hormone receptor status in primary and metastatic breast cancer. *Seminars in Oncology*, **12**(1), supplement 1, 12–16.

Padmanabhan, N., Howell, A. and Rubens, R.D. (1986) Mechanism of action of adjuvant chemotherapy in early breast cancer. *The Lancet*, ii, 411–14.

Powles, T.J. (1983) The role of aromatase inhibitors in breast cancer. *Seminars in Oncology*, **10**, supplement 4, 4.

Sque, M. (1985) What's in a name? *Nursing Mirror*, **160**(8), 22.

Stewart, H.J. (1992) Scottish Cancer Trials Breast Group – The Scottish trial of adjuvant tamoxifen in node negative breast cancer. *Monogr. National Cancer Institute*, **11**, 117–20.

Vallis, K. and Waxman, J. (1988) Tumour Flare in Hormonal Therapy, in *Endocrine Management of Cancer; Volume 2 Contemporary Therapy* (ed. B. Stoll), Karger, Basle.

Voda, A. (1986) Menopause. *Annual Review of Nursing Research*, **4**, 55–75.

Webb, C. (1985) *Sexuality, Nursing and Health*, J. Wiley and Sons, Chichester.

Breast reconstruction | 9

Joanna M. Parker

Breast reconstruction may be described as the creation of a breast form using autogenous tissue, with or without the insertion of an implant, in a woman who has completely, or partially, lost her breast through surgery for breast cancer.

In recent years, the number of women undergoing breast reconstruction has increased. This may be the result of improved surgical techniques, more media coverage and a greater understanding of the psychological problems experienced by women following mastectomy (Morris, Greer and Hite, 1977; Maguire et al., 1978). It has been suggested that breast reconstruction may help to minimize the psychological sequelae and aid rehabilitation, particularly in women whose body image is very important to their self-esteem (Georgiade et al., 1985; Goin and Goin, 1982). As a result more doctors are offering breast reconstruction to their patients.

Psychological benefits have been demonstrated in several studies (Dean, Chelty and Forrest, 1983; Meyer and Ringberg, 1986). These include increased freedom with clothing, more rapid resumption of work and social activities after surgery, increased confidence in participating in sport and expressions of feeling 'whole' again. Some women believe breast reconstruction to have been essential to their ability to cope with having a mastectomy (Georgiade et al., 1985; Meyer 1986); Dinner (1985) states that breast reconstruction may enable some women to accept mastectomy as a treatment who would otherwise have found it intolerable. Such demonstrated benefits mean that breast reconstruction should no longer be regarded as a luxury operation. In recognition of this and the fact that mastectomy continues to be considered by many as the best treatment for large, central and multifocal breast cancers, the King's Fund consensus development conference statement on treatment for breast cancer (Kings Fund Forum, 1986) recommends:

The possibility of breast reconstructive surgery be discussed with all women in whom a significant loss of breast tissue will be necessary.

The proportion of women who would want to undergo breast reconstruction if it were offered to all is not known, but it is likely to be more than the current facilities could cope with. At present, there are few plastic surgeons and specialist breast surgeons performing breast reconstructions, hence many women are not made aware of the possibility of reconstruction. It is to be hoped that this may change in the future.

However, it should be noted that the studies indicating the benefits of breast reconstruction also show that psychosocial problems, such as anxiety and depression, continue to be experienced frequently. Women may still have difficulties adjusting to an altered body image and they must still come to terms with having breast cancer. Gilboa and co-workers (1990) found single women and those who had recently undergone adjuvant therapies were most at risk of psychological problems following breast reconstruction. Soloman (1986) writes of her own experience:

> As pleased as I am with the results of breast reconstruction my pleasure does not erase the pain of mastectomy.

It should therefore not be presumed that women who have breast reconstructive surgery require less support than those who do not. Nurses and other members of the multidisciplinary team have an important role to play in patient education, preparation and care during and after breast reconstruction.

THE SELECTION OF PATIENTS FOR BREAST RECONSTRUCTION

Health professionals may endeavour to assess a woman's suitability for breast reconstruction, but the final decision must rest with the patient. Only the woman who has lost, or is to lose, her breast is able to perceive what that loss means to her and whether breast reconstruction is likely to help her. Dean, Chelty and Forrest (1983) state:

> The decision about breast reconstruction can safely be left to the patient, who alone knows the importance of her own breast.

However, if a woman is to make the decision it is important that she be well informed about what a breast reconstruction would involve for her, and that she has realistic expectations.

Advancing age and the presence of metastatic disease are frequently considered to be contra-indications, but this should not necessarily be so. Older women are often presumed to be less distressed by mutilating surgery than younger women and hence not to want, or not to need, breast reconstruction. But some elderly women are devastated at the loss of their breast and gain just as much benefit from breast reconstruction as younger women. Also, although uncontrolled or advanced metastatic disease means breast reconstruction is inappropriate, many surgeons today will consider breast reconstruction for a woman with metastatic disease if she is well enough to undergo surgery and believes it will bring her increased quality of life, if only for a limited time.

Ideally, every woman should be treated as an individual and, provided she is well enough, be given the opportunity of undergoing reconstruction. Patient self-selection would seem to be the best selection method, providing that the patients are well informed as to what this involves and their expectations are realistic.

Studies indicate that women share similar motives for seeking reconstruction, namely eliminating the need for an external prosthesis, to improve self-confidence/self-esteem, to be able to wear all types of clothing, to feel physically whole again (Goldberg, 1984; Clifford, 1979; Scain 1985). Very few women have been found to see it as a way of solving other problems, such as improving their marriage or sexual relationship (Clifford, 1979; Goin and Goin, 1988). Where they do seek it for this reason it should be explained that reconstruction is unlikely to solve these problems and that counselling may be more appropriate.

THE TIMING OF BREAST RECONSTRUCTION

Breast reconstruction may be undertaken at the time of mastectomy (immediate reconstruction). Most breast reconstructions were delayed in the past, but now immediate reconstructions are frequently performed in the hope of sparing the women some of the possible psychological morbidity associated with mastectomy, as well as avoiding further hospitalization and general anaesthesia.

Concern that immediate reconstruction may hide the existence of recurrent disease in the breast and compromise survival has led some surgeons to recommend a delay of several years. However, Watts (1980) points out that fewer than 10% of women experience local recurrence following mastectomy meaning that 90% of women would wait needlessly. They found that the survival rate of women who had immediate reconstruction was the same as those who had not. Darden, Blanchard and Greenstreet (1982) and Georgiade *et al.* (1985) support this. In addition Georgiade and co-workers (1985) state that by putting the implant behind the chest wall muscles, soft tissue recurrences were more easily detectable. Delay in carrying out reconstruction may be recommended if there is a high risk of local recurrence because of factors such as cancer infiltrating the skin, inflammatory cancer, ulceration and the involvement of a large number of axillary nodes.

The benefit that women who have immediate reconstructions will be more critical of the result and less satisfied because they have not lived with a mastectomy is not borne out by research. Dean, Chelty and Forrest (1983) and Meyer (1986) found that the majority of women were very satisfied with immediate reconstruction and felt it was important in helping them cope with the loss of their breast. Dean, Chelty and Forrest (1983) found that they suffered less psychosocial morbidity than those who had had mastectomies only. The findings of Noone *et al.* (1985) and Stevens *et al.* (1985) were similar.

The best time for an individual woman to undergo breast reconstruction will depend on several factors: those relating to the disease, type, size, spread of the cancer; whether a reconstructive surgeon is available at the time of mastectomy; and, most importantly, how the woman feels. Some women may be unsure whether a reconstruction is what they want and hence they prefer to wait. Others may feel an immediate reconstruction is imperative for their ability to cope with a mastectomy.

METHODS OF BREAST RECONSTRUCTION

There are several different methods of breast reconstruction. Which one is most suitable for a particular woman will depend on factors such as her desires and expectations, the size of her breast, the type of mastectomy performed (i.e. simple, modified radical or radical), the conditions of the skin and muscle overlaying the chest wall, and the possible need for surgery to the remaining breast in order to attain symmetry.

The four most commonly performed methods of breast reconstruction are discussed below. All may be performed as immediate or delayed reconstruction; most require the insertion of an implant to achieve the size and shape of a breast.

There has been some concern recently about silicone implants and the possible harmful effects they may have in the body in the long term. A polyurethane-coated silicone implant has recently been withdrawn from the market following worries about the carcinogenic effects of the polyurethane.

In early 1992, the American Food and Drug Administration (FDA) temporarily suspended sales of all silicone implants while it investigated studies of their effects, particularly a possible link with auto-immune diseases. The FDA currently recommends that silicone implants are used only in women having reconstructive surgery following mastectomy and not in purely cosmetic breast augmentation surgery as research continues. To date, the UK Department of Health has made no similar suggestion and believes that no significant health risk has been identified for women having silicone implants.

Subpectoral reconstruction

This is a relatively simple surgical procedure in which a breast implant is placed beneath the pectoralis major and serratus antenor muscles, which cover the chest wall (Figure 9.1). The surrounding tissues are sutured to form a pocket for the implant and to minimize the possibility of upward or lateral movement.

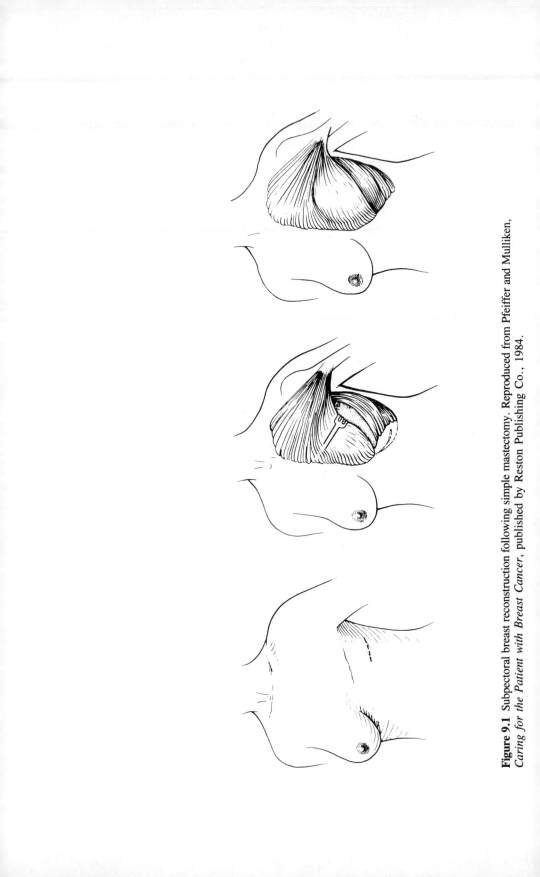

Figure 9.1 Subpectoral breast reconstruction following simple mastectomy. Reproduced from Pfeiffer and Mulliken, *Caring for the Patient with Breast Cancer*, published by Reston Publishing Co., 1984.

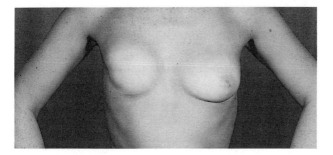

(a)

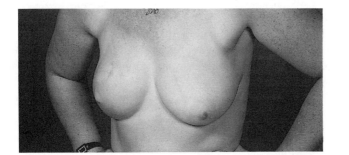

(b)

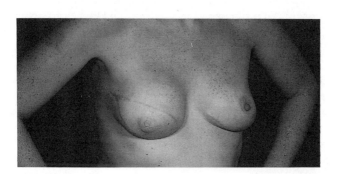

(c)

Figure 9.2 Subcutaneous reconstruction; (a) a young woman who had an immediate left breast reconstruction following a left simple mastectomy by subpectoral implant, (b) a woman who had a delayed left breast reconstruction using a Becker double lumien expander implant. She is also showing a stick-on silicone nipple and (c) a woman who had an immediate left breast reconstruction with a latissimus dorsi flap and a nipple reconstruction. She also had a right breast reduction to improve symmetry.

The breast reconstruction is performed through the same incision as the mastectomy, so there is no additional scarring. Unfortunately, this simple method achieves good results only if the woman has small breasts with little aptosis. It is not suitable for women who have had a radical mastectomy or if there has been severe radiation scarring.

Subcutaneous reconstruction

A subcutaneous reconstruction involves placing an implant beneath the skin of the breast following a subcutaneous mastectomy that has removed the breast tissue but preserved all the skin, areola and nipple (Figure 9.2). It is argued that this produces superior cosmetic results that are more acceptable to women (Art, Dinner and Sampliner, 1988). However, some studies indicate that long-term results are disappointing and complications are greater (Slade, 1984; Goldwyn and Goldman, 1976).

Furthermore, since it is impossible to remove all the breast tissue by subcutaneous mastectomy, many surgeons are concerned about the risk of recurrence in the preserved skin and nipple, and a total mastectomy is therefore often preferred. However, this method may be preferred for women seeking prophylactic mastectomy because of a strong family history of breast cancer.

Tissue expansion

This method is a three-stage procedure that makes use of the skin's ability to stretch (Figure 9.3). In an initial operation, an expandable implant, known as a tissue expander, is placed beneath the chest wall muscles. The tissue expander consists of a silicone sac with a port and valve through which saline can be injected to increase its size. At the time of the operation it is partially filled with saline to the degree allowed by the overlying tissue. Inflation proceeds at weekly or fortnightly intervals once the wound is considered to be sufficiently healed. The woman must attend as an out-patient for saline to be injected via the port, which is subcutaneous and lateral or medial to the expander. Expansion continues until a size greater than the other breast is achieved, which may take a few weeks or a few months.

The woman may experience discomfort, lasting for up to 48 hours, with each injection of saline as the skin and muscle is stretched. If it is found to be very painful, saline can be removed and the expansion proceeded with more slowly.

The second stage of the procedure is a period of over-expansion that lasts for at least three months so as to ensure permanent stretching of the tissue.

The third stage is the deflation and removal of the expander in a second operation, during which an implant of a size to match the womans own breast is placed *in situ*.

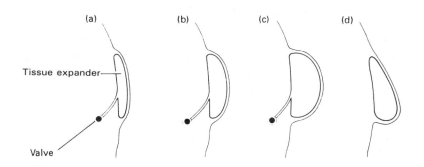

Figure 9.3 Tissue expansion; (a) immediately after surgery, (b) partly inflated, (c) over-expanded and (d) deflated with the valve removed. Reproduced from The Patient Education Group, *Breast Reconstruction*, published by The Royal Marsden Hospital, 1990.

At least six months is usually required for this method of breast reconstruction to be completed. However, it will depend on the rate at which inflation can occur and the size of the woman's breast. Sometimes it is possible to fully inflate the expander at the time of surgery but this depends on the amount and quality of skin and muscle overlaying it. Where the skin cover is limited, or the skin quality is poor – following radiotherapy for example – expansion must proceed more slowly. Too rapid expansion may compromise the circulation of the tissue and lead to necrosis and extrusion of the expander.

The period of over-expansion is important for two reasons. Firstly, stretching the skin and muscle beyond what is needed to accommodate the final implant creates a degree of ptosis and hence a more natural and symmetrical breast form. Secondly, over-expansion for a period of several months is thought to reduce the rate of severe capsular contractures forming.

A double lumen tissue expander is now available. The outer lumen contains silicone and the inner is the expander that can be filled with saline. Expansion proceeds in the same way, but this expander does not require removal. After the period of over-expansion, enough saline is withdrawn to equalize the size of the breasts. When the woman is satisfied that the size is right, the port is removed under local anaesthetic.

Tissue expansion is used where the skin is of good quality but inadequate quantity for subpectoral implant. It also enables greater symmetry to be achieved where a degree of ptosis is required and does not result in any additional scarring. Tissue expansion is not suitable following a radical mastectomy unless used with a myocutaneous flap. It can be used following radiotherapy, but expansion is usually slow and there may be difficulty attaining the required size if fibrosis in the skin and muscle is severe.

Myocutaneous flap breast reconstruction

Where the breast to be reconstructed is large or where the skin or muscle overlying the chest wall is inadequate, damaged by radiotherapy or missing following a radical mastectomy, breast reconstruction using tissue expansion or a subpectoral implant is not generally possible. Reconstruction using a myocutaneous flap (an area of skin and muscle from another part of the body) is then the method of choice. The two common sites for myocutaneous flaps used in breast reconstruction are the latissimus dorsi muscle of the back and the rectus abdominis muscle of the abdomen.

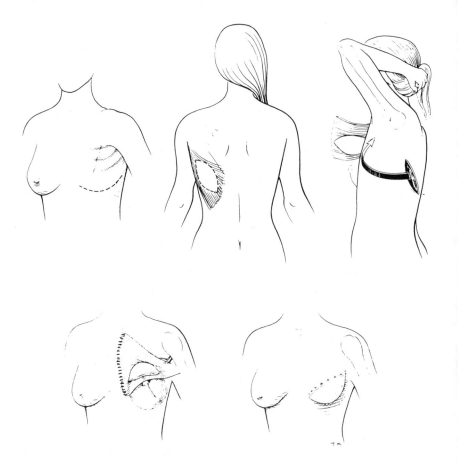

Figure 9.4 Stages of the latissimus dorsi myocutaneous flap. Reproduced from Pfeiffer and Mulliken, *Caring for the Patient with Breast Cancer*, published by Reston Publishing Co., 1984.

Latissimus dorsi myocutaneous flap

The latissimus dorsi is a large flat muscle. It arises from the lower six vertebrae, the lumbar fascia and the crest of ileum and inserts into the bicipital groove of the humerus. The majority of the muscle lies subcutaneously and is therefore easily accessible to the surgeon.

When used in breast reconstruction, part of the latissimus dorsi muscle and an area of overlying skin and its blood supply are dissected, rotated on a pedicle and tunnelled beneath the skin under the arm to lie on the anterior chest wall. Here it is used to cover the implant and joined to the skin and muscle already there. Occasionally, if the breast to be reconstructed is very small, an implant is not required. The donor site on the back is sutured to form a horizontal or oblique scar.

Figure 9.4 shows a latissimus dorsi flap reconstruction and demonstrates the scarring that results both on the breast and on the back. The latissimus dorsi flap is versatile and allows a large area of muscle to be transported without causing functional disabilities for most women. Tissue deficits in the clavicular and axillary regions can also be partially rectified using this flap. Functional disabilities can result if the nerve to the latissimus dorsi is damaged during surgery.

Rectus abdominis myocutaneous flap

The rectus abdomini is a long flap muscle that runs from the pubis to the costal cartilages of the fifth, sixth and seventh ribs. It is one of the superficial muscles of the abdominal wall supplied by the superior and deep epigastric arteries.

A transverse or vertical portion of the muscle can be used for breast reconstruction, but as the former leaves a less obtrusive scar it is often preferred (Figure 9.5). An area of muscle and skin with its blood supply is rotated and passed through a subcutaneous tunnel on to the chest wall where it is fashioned into the shape of a breast. It can also be usd as a free flap but this requires microsurgery for it to remain viable and is therefore less common. The donor site on the abdomen is closed to form a single scar, but first a supportive mesh is usually inserted to strengthen the abdominal wall and reduce the risk of herniation.

This method of breast reconstruction allows a large amount of tissue to be transposed, so it is often possible to avoid the use of an implant. This removes the risk of capsular contracture and gives a more natural feel to the breast. Skin from the abdomen may provide a better colour and texture match than that provided by the latissimus dorsi muscle.

Despite the advantages of the rectus abdominis flap it is used less frequently than other methods of reconstruction, partly because it requires a longer period of convalescence for the patient. It is therefore used when other methods

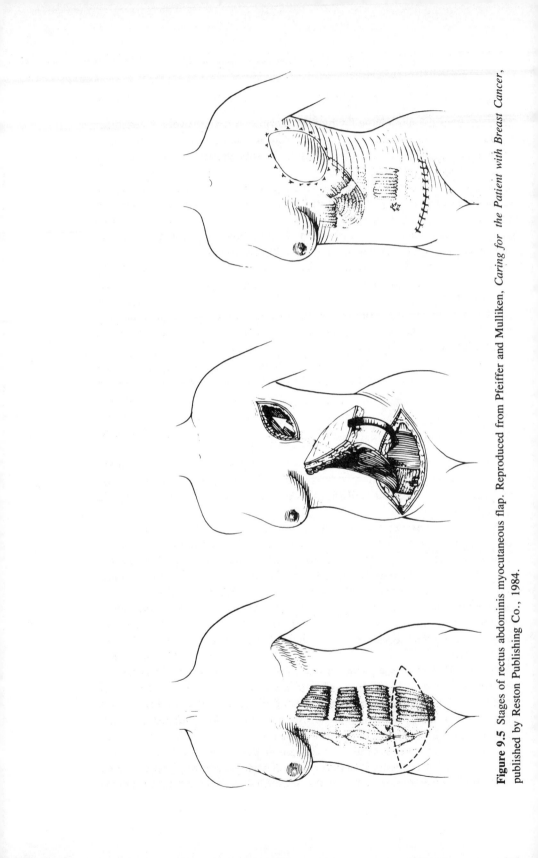

Figure 9.5 Stages of rectus abdominis myocutaneous flap. Reproduced from Pfeiffer and Mulliken, *Caring for the Patient with Breast Cancer,* published by Reston Publishing Co., 1984.

are not considered suitable. Lerberg and Prin (1991) suggest it is particularly useful when the latissimus dorsi muscle is divided or atrophic, if there have been previous problems with silicone implants, if a woman has very large breasts or if there are large defects in the axillary or intraclavicular region. It should be avoided or used with caution in patients where microcirculation may be diminished, such as women who are obese, have diabetes or are smokers, or where there has been previous surgery or radiotherapy to the area of the flap or its blood supply.

SURGERY TO THE OPPOSITE BREAST

Surgery to the opposite breast is frequently required if the greatest degree of symmetry between the breasts is to be achieved. This may involve the reduction of a large breast, augmentation of a small breast or surgery to reduce the ptosis of a very pendulous breast.

Although many women do want symmetrical breasts, some prefer a degree of asymmetry to having to undergo additional surgery involving their other breast. In agreeing to surgery of this nature the woman should be aware of what is involved, the scarring that results and the possible loss of nipple sensation in that breast. Also the 'cancer status' of this breast must be considered because surgery will cause scarring which may make subsequent clinical and mammographic assessment difficult.

NIPPLE-AREOLAR RECONSTUCTION

Preservation of the nipple in women undergoing mastectomy and breast reconstruction is considered inadvisable because of the risk of recurrent disease developing in the preserved nipple. Bishop, Singh and Nash (1990) suggest that women undergoing mastectomy and breast reconstruction for a recurrence of cancer in a breast previously treated by lumpectomy and radiotherapy are suitable for nipple preservation providing the tumour is 3 cm from the nipple. This is a small but significant group of women. The majority will continue to have the nipple removed as part of mastectomy.

Reconstruction of the nipple areolar complex is possible, however. It is usually carried out several months after completion of the breast reconstruction to allow the breast to 'settle'. The most common method is to use the skin and fat of the reconstructed breast to create the nipple and then to take a full thickness skin graft from the inner thigh to form the areola. Tattooing may be used to obtain a better colour match (Becker, 1986). Skin from the ear and labia have also been used but are generally less acceptable to the woman.

A study in The Netherlands suggests that large numbers of women want reconstrution of the nipple aerolar complex: 56% of those in a study by Haupt,

Dykstra and von Leenwen (1988) wanted this carried out. Fewer women seem to undergo the procedure in the UK, although the reasons for this are unclear. Many women prefer to use adhesive silicone nipples or to have none at all.

NURSING MANAGEMENT OF WOMEN UNDERGOING SURGERY FOR BREAST RECONSTRUCTION

The role of caring for women undergoing breast reconstruction falls largely to nurses working both in hospitals and in the community. They are in an ideal position to support women and their families before, during and after the hospital stay, but in order to do this effectively nurses need a sound base of knowledge about breast cancer and its management as well as breast reconstruction. In addition, they need to have developed communication skills so as to be better able to identify and meet the needs of the women in their care.

Pre-admission

Nursing management begins when a woman first visits the hospital to discuss breast reconstruction with her surgeon. Between this visit and when she is admitted to hospital for surgery, nurses have an important supportive and educational role to play in helping a woman to clarify her feelings about breast reconstruction and providing her with the information she requires to decide whether to have the procedure. This can be a very difficult decision to make, particularly if she is coming to terms with a recent diagnosis of breast cancer and the prospect of mastectomy, or is experiencing the shock and disappointment of local recurrence of cancer following previous conservative surgery. The needs of such women may be very different from those of women seeking delayed reconstruction several years after a mastectomy. Nurses must therefore be sensitive in their assessment of an individual's needs and flexible in their approach to care.

Assessment

Assessment at this time should include ascertaining how a woman feels about having breast cancer and how it is affecting her life and that of her family. This may reveal areas of anxiety – fears about death and dying, cancer recurrence and the effects of treatments such as chemotherapy and radiotherapy. It is particularly important for the women considering immediate reconstruction.

How a woman feels about having had a mastectomy or the prospect of losing her breast should also be discussed. This will encourage the expression and exploration of feelings while enabling the nurse to assess the woman's body image and self-esteem, how she perceives her femininity and sexuality, and how these may be affected. The nurse may thus be able to identify the women who will be particularly helped by breast reconstruction.

It is important for the nurse to assess the level of knowledge the woman has. This will allow her to identify the areas of information needed to enable the woman to decide whether to have a breast reconstruction and to ensure that consent is truly 'informed'. Some women may have read extensively, seen television programmes or know someone who has had a breast reconstruction. Others may have almost no knowledge at all. The nurse should also clarify how much information the woman has received from other health care professionals about the operation, the likely post-operative experience and possible complications, and whether the woman has understood it correctly. Where possible, the nurse should be present during the consultation with the surgeon so she knows what was said and can more easily evaluate how much the woman was able to take in.

The woman's motives for and expectations of breast reconstruction should also be ascertained. It is possible that women who undergo reconstruction for themselves rather than for others have a more realistic expectation as to what the reconstructed breast will look like and how it may improve their quality of life, and are possibly more likely to be satisfied with the outcome of breast reconstruction.

Three other areas that should be assessed are the woman's social support system and mental health state, and any concurrent stresses in her life. Research has suggested that single women, those with previous psychiatric illness and those with other areas of stress in their lives – such as divorce, unemployment, or the death or serious illness of someone close to them – are more likely to have psychosocial problems following the diagnosis and treatment of breast cancer (Morris, Greer and Hite, 1977; Denton and Baum, 1983). By identifying those with a higher risk, the nurse can offer additional support where appropriate, refer the woman to support agencies and/or observe them more closely in the post-operative period.

Physical assessment will be more thoroughly undertaken on admission to hospital, but in the pre-admission period the nurse should be aware of any specific health problems the patient has. She should also find out what previous breast surgery has been undertaken; whether the skin and muscles of the chest wall are in good condition and whether there has been any radiotherapy to that area or the donor site of a myocutaneous flap.

Patient education

The aim of patient education is to enable the woman to decide whether to have breast reconstruction surgery, to prepare her for that surgery and to help her adjust after it. Women vary in the amount of information they want. Most are eager to understand what breast reconstruction involves, but some wish for very little information and this must be respected.

The nurse should discuss the proposed method of reconstruction outlining what the operation involves and the likely post-operative experience, including the presence of wound drains, intravenous infusions, pain and the extent of scarring.

Where tissue expansion is being used the woman should be made aware of how long it will take to complete the reconstruction and the fact that some women find this frustrating. She must also be told that she will need to attend hospital frequently for inflation of the prosthesis and that each inflation may cause discomfort. In addition she must understand that during the period of over-expansion the breast may be markedly asymmetrical, requiring the use of a temporary prosthesis to build up the size of her natural breast to achieve symmetry.

Potential early and late complications should be explored with the woman (Table 9.1), particularly the possibility of post-operative infection and the risk of capsular contracture developing that may require removal of the implant. Some women are very concerned about the possible effects of silicone implants in their bodies.

Table 9.1 Early and late complications of breast reconstruction

Early	Late
Haematoma	Capsular contracture
Seroma	Extrusion of prosthesis
Infection	Reduced shoulder function
Necrosis	Abdominal herniation
Tissue expander valve failure	Asymmetry
Paraesthesia arm/chest wall	

Giving information about the appearance of a breast reconstruction helps to promote realistic expectations. This can be done most effectively by drawings and photographs. Most women find these helpful but a few prefer not to see any. Where possible photographs of reconstructions performed by the surgeon who is to do the woman's operation should be used. These should not be confined to the best results that might be attained as there is no guarantee of the outcome. Sometimes women may wish to see an example of the implant that will be used.

Many women also find it helpful to talk to someone who has undergone a similar operation. It is useful to maintain a list of women willing to be contacted for such a purpose, but if the nurse does not know anyone who is suitable, Breast Cancer Care (formerly the Breast Care and Mastectomy Association) may be able to put the woman in touch with a volunteer who has had similar surgery.

Where appropriate, the nurse should discuss the possibility of surgery to the opposite breast. It should be made clear that the aim is to attain a more symmetrical appearance but that it does result in scarring of this breast and may cause the loss of nipple sensation.

A tremendous amount of information is usually given to a woman considering breast reconstruction. While she may actively want it, it may be very difficult to assimilate it all in one session. It is often helpful for her partner or a friend or relative to be present, but it is important that she is given the opportunity to return to talk to the surgeon or clinical nurse specialist at a later date. Where possible a contact telephone number should be given, and the nurse should encourage each woman to note down questions that occur to her at home to bring to the next consultation.

A decision to undergo breast reconstruction should not be made hastily and a woman needs the nurse's time to go over the information she has been given. An information booklet that she can take home is useful as an *aide-mémoire* for information given verbally, and the woman may like to share this with her family to help them understand what is involved.

Psychological support

By being available to listen to what a woman has to say and encourage her to express and explore her feelings the nurse is able to demonstrate caring and provide support. This supportive role may extend to other members of the woman's family; indeed, where this occurs support for the woman is likely to be more effective. Many women find having a telephone contact number a very important and practical means of support. The nurse may also find that she is required to act as a patient advocate, by presenting the woman's concerns or views to the doctors, or by giving her moral support to do this herself.

Pre-operatively

Once a woman has decided to undergo reconstruction and has been admitted to hospital, a more formal nursing assessment will be completed. Ideally, the same nurse would continue the assessment begun before admission, but this is rarely possible so the areas mentioned previously will have to be reassessed and any new fears or concerns identified.

Further discussion of the operation may be required, and the nurse should ensure that the woman understands what is to happen to her and that informed consent has been obtained by the doctor. Discussion of the appearance of the surgical wounds may be helpful at this time. Knowing that bruising and the presence of suture material affect the appearance of the reconstructed breast may avoid the woman being shocked when she first looks at her scars. Looking at the reconstruction for the first time is often difficult, particularly if it is an immediate reconstruction following mastectomy. To look down at a small area of the breast initially may lessen the trauma. It is usually a good idea for a woman to get used to looking at the reconstruction from above before looking in the mirror, but she should be encouraged to do this when she feels able.

Post-operative nursing management

Following the woman's return to the ward the nurse should take her temperature, pulse and blood pressure and observe the surgical wounds and wound drains, gradually decreasing the frequency from quarter-hourly to half-hourly to four-hourly if her condition remains stable. The frequency of observations is individually determined according to the patient's progress.

Usually at least two closed wound drains are inserted into the area of the reconstructed breast. They should be observed for patency and to ensure that there is no evidence of haemorrhage, of which there is a greater risk following immediate reconstruction because of the removal of the breast and axillary lymph nodes. Drains usually remain *in situ* for 3–5 days until wound drainage is minimal. Wound drains reduce the risk of haematoma and seroma formations but if left *in situ* too long may increase the risk of infection.

Excessive bleeding may not always be apparent from observing the wound drains but may be detected by bleeding from the wound itself or by a sudden increase in the size of the breast as a result of haematoma formation. Transparent dressings are often used to allow the nurse to observe the surgical wounds frequently. Small haematomas are not uncommon, particularly following immediate reconstruction, and they are absorbed by the body in time. Large haematomas may require surgical evacuation and occasionally necessitate removal of the implant.

Surgical wounds should also be observed to detect signs of inadequate blood perfusion. This is particularly important where myocutaneous flaps have been used. Survival of the flap depends primarily on the maintenance of its blood supply. If this is damaged during or after surgery part or all of the flap may die, but early detection of problems may enable surgical revision.

The nurse should observe the flaps for colour, temperature and capillary refill. Normally it is pale pink in colour; a dusky pink or bluish colour could indicate venous congestion, which may eventually lead to necrosis. The skin of the flap should feel warm to the touch; if it is cooler than the surrounding tissues it may indicate a problem with blood perfusion.

Capillary refill can be assessed by applying gentle pressure to the flap with a finger. If perfusion is good the tissue will blanch but the colour will return again within a few seconds; if it does not the cause is very likely to be venous congestion.

Tight dressings and the application of any pressure should be avoided as this may interfere with circulation within the flap. The incidence of necrosis is fortunately low. It is more common following the use of myocutaneous flaps, but can occur with any method of reconstruction. Haupt, Dykstra and von Leenwen reported that only 1 out of 72 women experienced partial loss of a latissimus dorsi flap as a result of necrosis, and Hartrumpf and Bennett (1987) reported 6% partial loss and 1% total loss of rectus flap. The incidence of flap necrosis was higher in heavy smokers.

The nurse must also observe the wound for signs of infection: discharge, erythema, tenderness or increased temperature. This is particularly important in breast reconstruction surgery since infection may compromise the viability of the myocutaneous flap or necessitate removal of the implant. To reduce this risk prophylactic antibiotics may be prescribed.

If an infection does occur the implant can become the focus of it, which may be difficult to manage. Obviously, asepsis in changing dressings and wound drains is very important and dressings should only be changed if it is essential to do so.

Fortunately, persistent infection requiring the removal of an implant or causing the failure of part of a myocutaneous flap is rare. Georgiade et al. (1985) reported that the implant had to be removed because of infection in 1% of cases.

Post-operative discomfort following surgery for breast reconstruction varies according to the method used and the individual patient. Women undergoing immediate reconstruction who are also having axillary dissection, and those having a rectus abdominis myocutaneous flap (and hence an abdominal wound) are likely to experience the most discomfort. Most women require regular analgesia for approximately four days, but generally only require opiate analgesia for the first 24 hours. Women undergoing reconstruction via rectus abdominis myocutaneous flaps may particularly benefit from having continuous analgesic infusions during this period. Analgesia may be required before physiotherapy exercises for a more prolonged period.

Discharge preparation

In preparation for discharge from hospital any concerns the woman has about going home should be discussed. Many women are worried that something may happen to the wounds or implant. It is advisable to give a contact number, e.g. for the ward or clinical nurse specialist, so that the woman can telephone about any problems or anxieties that she has. She should be aware of the problems that can arise, such as development of a seroma (particularly if there has been axillary node dissection) or wound infection, and that medical advice should be sought if this occurs.

Some surgeons advise massage of the reconstructed breast following removal of the sutures in the belief that this may reduce fibrous tissue formation and hence reduce the incidence of capsular contractures; but there is no research to support this theory. However, some women do find gently rubbing in a simple unperfumed moisturizing cream to be soothing, particularly those undergoing tissue expansion. This will also encourage a woman to touch her reconstructed breast, which may be of psychological benefit in helping her to incorporate it into her body image. It should be explained to her that the reconstruction may feel quite hard and swollen in the first few weeks after surgery and may take two or three months to soften. It will, however, always feel different from her natural breast.

In the first two months after surgery a supportive bra is usually the most comfortable. Sports or dance bras, which are very supportive and have fewer seams, are preferred by some. The nurse should be able to give advice on bras that are suitable for wearing following a reconstruction. Some surgeons prefer women to wear special support jackets, particularly following latissimus dorsi myocutaneous flap, to prevent the implant from migrating. Once the reconstruction has settled down any form of bra may be worn, or none at all if that is preferred.

Discomfort, particularly when moving the arm, will continue for several weeks, gradually lessening. There is usually no sensation in the reconstructed breast, but phantom nipple sensations are not uncommon following mastectomy. Women should be told that these will go in time. Sometimes strange sensations are felt in the breast, referred from the back or abdomen following a myocutaneous flap. Again these will cease in time.

Women undergoing tissue expansion will require a temporary external prosthesis to be fitted to supplement the size of their reconstructed breast. The temporary prosthesis should be one from which filling can be removed so that the size can be adjusted as expansion proceeds. During the period of over-expansion it can be used to build up the natural breast so that symmetry can be maintained. The nurse should also give guidance about clothing that will minimize the appearance of asymmetry during over-expansion.

Silicone nipples are available and can be fitted as soon as the wounds are healed; they may be particularly necessary while wearing swimwear. Some women wear them on a long-term basis, others just until they have nipple reconstruction.

As is the case after other operations, many women who feel well in hospital may feel tired once they go home. Women should be warned that this is likely. However, they should be encouraged gradually to take up their social life again. When the women go back to work will depend on individual factors such as the type of work they do, whether adjuvant therapies are being given and the method of reconstruction, but many women are able to go back after about six weeks.

Nursing management following discharge from hospital

Breast care nurses, out-patient nurses, Macmillan nurses and district nurses may all be involved in seeing women who have had breast reconstruction.

The aim of management at this stage should be to provide psychological support, identify any problems in coping and offer practical advice to deal with any problems that occur.

The nurse should observe for signs of anxiety and depression, assessing the woman's feelings and mood, her appetite, sleep and social behaviour. She should ask her about her satisfaction with her appearance and how she really feels about her reconstruction. Assessing her relationship with her partner and whether he or she has seen her breast yet may help the nurse to judge how supportive her home situation is and if any additional stresses are being experienced. If anxiety, depression or sexual problems are evident the nurse should, with the woman's consent, make a referral to an appropriate agency.

The nurse must also be aware of the possible later complications of breast reconstruction (Table 9.1). The most common of these is capsular contracture. This occurs when the body reacts to the breast implant by producing fibrous tissue to seal it in a capsule. Over time this tissue contracts and may cause discomfort, hardness of the breast and an alteration in shape. It may be possible for the surgeon to break the capsule by applying manual pressure. More commonly, surgery is required to break or remove the capsule and replace the implant.

The incidence of capsular contracture is difficult to ascertain because a certain degree is present whenever an implant is used, although it is not usually severe enough to cause problems. Estimated and reported rates of contractures vary from 0% (Artz, Dinner and Sampliner, 1988) to 60% (Ward, 1987).

Rates of severe contracture tend to be below 10%. Gibney (1987) reports 5.8% following tissue expansion and subpectoral implant, Schuster and Lavine (1988) report 4% severe enough to warrant the removal of the implant following tissue expansion and subpectoral implant; Goin and Goin (1988) report an overall rate of 25%; while Haupt, Dykstra and von Leenwen (1988) report no severe contractures (grade 4 Baker scale), but moderate capsular contracture (Grade 3 Baker scale) rates of 5% following latissimus dorsi flap and 14% following subpectoral implants.

Companies that manufacture implants are constantly trying to reduce the incidence of capsular contractures using new technology. Recent findings by Coleman, Foo and Sharpe (1991) suggest textured implants may significantly reduce it.

Other potential complications include extrusion of the tissue expander. This occurs mainly in women who have poor quality skin and have had previous radiotherapy; it is therefore most important that the surgeon makes a careful assessment of the woman's skin pre-operatively so as to avoid the distress extrusion causes. When it does occur removal of the expander is necessary and reconstruction with a myocutaneous flap is required.

Deflation of the expander as a result of valve failure or accidental puncture during inflation is another problem that may occur. Schuster and Lavine (1988) reported 10%, Gibney (1987) reported 4.5%.

If any of these complications do occur it will cause the woman distress and disappointment even if she was aware of the possibility. She is likely to require a lot of support from the nurse as she considers whether to undergo further attempts at reconstruction.

Abdominal herniation has been discussed as a possible complication following rectus abdominis surgery. Hartrumpf and Bennett (1987) reported herniation in 2.9% of patients.

Impaired shoulder movement may occur following breast reconstruction, particularly when the axilla has undergone dissection or a latissimus dorsi flap has been raised. Physiotherapy may lessen or avert this problem. Nurses should observe how a woman is moving her arm and shoulder. Where there is impairment she should arrange for physiotherapy assessment. Early action is likely to prevent long-term problems.

The other main area of concern is whether it meets the woman's expectations or not. Most studies indicate women are happy to have undergone breast reconstructive surgery (Dean, Chelty and Forrest, 1983; Haupt, Dykstra and von Leenwen, 1988; Meyer and Bingberg, 1986) and would undergo it again even if they felt results were poorer than expected (Asplund 1984; Haupt, Dykstra and von Leenwen, 1988). A few women are dissatisfied, however. Meyer and Ringberg (1986) found these women tended to be characterized by high ambition, orderliness, high self-confidence, obstinacy and compulsion. Satisfaction was not affected by the number of complications or the need for further surgery.

One reason for dissatisfaction is asymmetry. The reconstructed breast may be slightly higher, smaller and have less ptosis than the woman's natural breast. In a bra the symmetry may be good, but if there is a noticeable difference a partial external prosthesis may help to attain a more balanced appearance. If a woman is dissatisfied with reconstruction the nurse should ask her to define again what her expectations had been and endeavour to find out if there are any other problems, e.g. marital, sexual or with body image, that may be influencing this dissatisfaction.

SUMMARY

Breast reconstruction may enable some women to cope more easily with having a mastectomy. It should be discussed with all women who are going to have a mastectomy since only they can assess accurately whether it would be of benefit to them. It may be performed as an immediate or delayed procedure by submuscular implants, tissue expansion or myocutaneous flap techniques. Nipple areolar complex reconstruction may also be performed at a later date, and surgery to the contralateral breast may be undertaken to attain symmetry.

The nurse has a very important role to play in supporting the woman and her family throughout this experience, beginning before her admission to hospital and continuing beyond discharge home.

Pre-operative care should include assessment of the motives, expectations and knowledge of breast reconstruction, and provision of the information a woman needs when deciding whether to have breast reconstructive surgery. The promotion of realistic expectations is particularly important if the woman is to be satisfied with the outcome of reconstruction. In order to do this, and to provide a high standard of nursing care during the hospital stay and beyond, the nurse must have a sound knowledge of breast reconstructive surgery procedures, the early and late complications that can occur and the potential psychological problems experienced by women who have undergone reconstruction. The nurse must also work to ensure good communications are maintained within the multidisciplinary team, while being prepared to act as the patient's advocate where necessary.

REFERENCES

Artz, J.S., Dinner, M.I., Sampliner, J. (1988) Breast reconstruction with subcutaneous tissue expander, followed with a polyurethane covered silicone implant. *Annals of Plastic Surgery*, vol **20**, 6, 587.

Asplund, O. and Karloff, B. (1984) Late results following mastectomy for cancer and breast reconstruction. *Scandinavian Journal of Plastic Reconstructive Surgery*, **18**, 221–5.

Becker, H. (1986) The use of intradermal tattoo to enhance the final result of nipple areolar reconstruction. *Plastic Reconstructive Surgery*, **77**, 673–75.

Bishop, C.C.R., Singh, S. and Nash, A.G. (1990) Mastectomy and breast reconstruction preserving the nipple. *Annals of the Royal College of Surgeons of England*, **72**, 87–9.

Clifford, E. (1979) The Reconstructive Experience – The Search For Restitution, in *Breast Reconstruction Following Mastectomy* (ed. N.G. Georgiade), CV Mosby, St Louis, Missouri.

Coleman, D.J., Foo, I.T.H. and Sharpe, D.T. (1991) Textured or smooth implants for breast augmentation? A prospective controlled trial. *British Journal of Plastic Surgery*, **44**, 444–8.

Dean, A., Chelty, N. and Forrest, A.P.M. (1983) Effects of immediate breast reconstruction on psychological morbidity after mastectomy. *The Lancet*, 26 Feb, 459–62.

Dowden, R.V., Blanchard, J.M. and Greenstreet, R.L. (1982) Breast reconstruction: selection, timing and local recurrence. *Annals of Plastic Surgery*, **10**, 265–9.

Denton, S. and Baum, M. (1983) Psychological Aspects of Breast Cancer, in *Breast Cancer* (ed. R. Margolese), Churchill Livingstone, Edinburgh.

Dinner, M.S. (1984) Post mastectomy reconstruction. *Surgical Clinics North America*, **64**(6), 1193–1207.

Dinner, M.I. and Coleman, C. (1985) Breast reconstruction. Use of autogenous tissue. *Association of Registered Nurses Journal*, **42**(4), 490–6.

Georgiade, G.S., Riefkolul, R., Cox, E., *et al.* (1985) Long term clinical outcome of immediate reconstruction after mastectomy. *Plastic Reconstructive Surgery*, **76**, 415.

Gibney, J. (1987) The long term results of tissue expansion for breast reconstruction. *Clinical Plastic Surgery*, **14** 509–18.

Gilboa, D., Borenstein, A., Floro, S. *et al.* (1990) Emotional and psychological adjustment of women to breast reconstruction and detection of subgroups at risk for psychological morbidity. *Annals of Plastic Surgery*, **25**, 397–401.

Goin, M.K. and Goin, J.M. (1982) Psychological reactions to prophylactic mastectomy synchronous with contralateral breast reconstruction. *Plastic Reconstructive Surgery*, **70**, 355–9.

Goin, M.K. and Goin, J.M. (1988) Growing pains: the psychological experience of breast reconstruction with tissue expansion. *Annals of Plastic Surgery*, **21**(3).

Goldberg, P., Stolzman, M., Goldberg, H.M. (1984) Psychological considerations in breast reconstruction. *Annals of Plastic Surgery*, **13**(38).

Goldwyn, R.M. and Goldman, L.D. (1976) Subcutaneous Mastectomies and Breast Replacement, in *Plastic and Reconstructive Surgery of the Breast* (ed. R.M. Goldwyn), Little & Brown, Boston, MA.

Hartrumpf, C.J. and Bennett, K.G. (1987) Autogenous tissue reconstruction in the mastectomy patient: a critical review. *Annals of Surgery*, **205**, 108–19.

Haupt, P., Dykstra, R. and von Leenwen, J.B.S. (1988) The result of breast reconstruction after mastectomy for breast cancer in 109 patients. *Annals of Plastic Surgery*, **121**(6), 517–25.

King's Fund Forum (1986) Consensus development conference: treatment of primary breast cancer. *British Medical Journal*, **293**, 946–7.

Lerberg, L. and Prin, J. (1991) T.R.A.M. Breast reconstruction. *Plastic Surgical Nursing*, **11**(2), 58–61.

Maguire, P., Lee., E.G., Bevington, D.J. *et al.* (1978) Psychiatric problems in the first year after mastectomy. *British Medical Journal*, 15 April, 963–5.

Maguire, P. *et al.* (1983) The effect of counselling on physical disability and social recovery after mastectomy. *Clinical Oncology*, **9**, 319–24.

Meyer, L. and Ringberg, A. (1986) A prospective study of psychiatric and psychosocial sequelae of bilateral subcutaneous mastectomy. *Scandinavian Journal of Plastic Reconstructive Sugery*, **20**, 101–7.

Morris, T., Greer, S. and Hite, P. (1977) Psychological and social adjustment to mastectomy: a two year follow up study. *Cancer*, **40**, 2381–7.

Noone, R.B., Murphy, J.B., Spear, S.L. and Little, J. VII (1985) A six year experience with immediate reconstruction after mastectomy for cancer. *Plastic Reconstructive Surgery*, **76**, 258–69.

Scain, W.S., Wellisch, D.K., Pasnan, R.O. and Landsvert, J. (1985) The sooner the better: a study of psychological factors in women undergoing immediate versus delayed breast reconstruction. *Annals of the Journal of Psychiatry* **142**, 40–6.

Schuster, D. and Lavine, D. (1988) A nine year experience with subpectoral breast reconstruction after subcutaneous mastectomy in 98 patients using saline inflatable prosthesis. *Annals of Plastic Surgery*, **21**(5), 444–51.

Slade, C.L. (1984) Subcutaneous mastectomy: acute complication and long term follow up. *Plastic Reconstructive Surgery*, **73**, 84–8.

Soloman, J. (1986) The good news about breast reconstruction. *Registered Nurse*, November, 47–54.

Stevens, L.A., McGrath, M.H., Russ, R.G. *et al.* (1985) The psychological impact of immediate reconstruction for women with early breast cancer. *Plastic Reconstructive Surgery*, **73**, 619–26.

Ward, D.J. (1987) Breast reconstruction. *Hospital Update*. September, 725.

Watts, G.T. *et al.* (1980) Mastectomy with primary reconstruction. *The Lancet*, **2**, 967.

Prosthetics | 10

Joanna M. Parker

The diagnosis of breast cancer is a devastating experience for most women. They have to face not only a potentially life-threatening illness, but also the possibility of mutilating surgery. For the majority of women the main initial concern is likely to be adequate treatment of the breast cancer, but most will also be worried about the partial or complete loss of their breast; for some this will be paramount (Denton and Baum, 1983; Maguire *et al.*, 1978). The psychological sequelae of the diagnosis and treatment of breast cancer are described in Chapter 2.

Restoring a woman's breast contour after surgery is a very important part of aiding her in her endeavours to adjust to the diagnosis and her altered body image. It may be achieved either by providing an external prosthesis, to be worn inside a bra, or by surgical breast reconstruction. External prostheses remain the most common method of restoring breast contours after partial or complete mastectomy, but there has recently been an increase in the number of women undergoing breast reconstruction.

EXTERNAL BREAST PROSTHESES

An external breast prosthesis is a false breast form that can be placed inside a bra. The aim is to enable a woman to attain an equal and balanced appearance when dressed following the partial or complete loss of her breast.

A soft, temporary prosthesis should be fitted a few days after surgery to be worn until the wound is well healed. A heavier, more realistic breast form (permanent prosthesis) can usually be fitted six to eight weeks after surgery or two weeks after the completion of radiotherapy when the skin is well healed.

Many women who have lost a breast experience feelings of vulnerability and a loss of attractiveness, femininity or sexuality. Providing a closely matching prosthesis is an essential part of aiding the rehabilitation of such a woman. It may encourage her to feel more confident in taking up her normal social life again and to believe that the loss of her breast is not obvious to everyone she meets. It may also help her to come to terms with her altered body image and re-establish her self-esteem. It is therefore essential that every woman has access to a prosthetic service delivered by a skilled practitioner who is able to give advice on prosthetics and clothing.

At present there is very little information about the quality of prosthetic services, but Simpson's survey (1985) suggests they are variable and often inadequate. In this study 32 prosthetic fitters and 92 patients from different parts of the UK were interviewed. Many patients were unhappy with the service they had received: 30% had never received a temporary prosthesis, and 50% of those who had had not had it fitted; 46% were unhappy with the permanent prosthesis, describing it as too heavy, not fitting properly or disliking the look and feel; 67% were only shown one permanent prosthesis, and in 65% of cases the fitting took less than 15 minutes. Fitting premises lacked privacy, were often cramped and did not have a mirror.

Interestingly, 61% of patients felt the attitude of the fitter contributed most to their dissatisfaction with the service. Fitters were appliance officers, orthotists, clinical nurse specialists and company representatives. Clinical nurse specialists fared well in the patients' evaluations and it can be argued that incorporating prosthetic fitting into a specialist nurse role increases the continuity of care for the patients and provides the nurse with an opportunity to assess the woman's physical and psychological well-being following her surgery.

TEMPORARY PROSTHESES

Several different types of temporary prostheses exist. They vary in size and shape (see Figure 10.1) but most consist of a cotton or nylon outer cover filled with a soft artificial lambswool material. All women who have lost a significant amount of their breast tissue should have a temporary prosthesis fitted into their bra prior to leaving hospital. Some women may prefer to have one pinned inside their nightdress immediately after their return from theatre and before the arrival of visitors. Table 10.1 shows information that should be given to patients about temporary prostheses.

Simpson's survey (1985) suggests little time and effort is given to the fitting of a temporary prosthesis, yet it is with this that the woman must first face the outside world. It is essential, therefore, that time is taken to fit the prosthesis and to show the woman how to position it within her bra. Because of its lightness, symmetry may be difficult to achieve, particularly where the remaining breast is large and heavy. The wearing of looser clothing until the permanent prosthesis is fitted can be suggested to women having this problem.

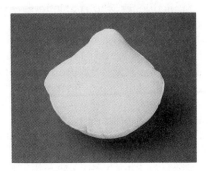

Figure 10.1 A temporary prosthesis.

Table 10.1 Information for patients about temporary prostheses

---

- Show how to position the prosthesis in the bra, adjusting the bra straps to accommodate for the lack of weight of the prosthesis.

- Discuss the use of safety pins and press-studs, and the benefits of stitching the prosthesis to secure it in the bra to prevent movement.

- Discuss the use of loose clothing when wearing a temporary prosthesis if symmetry between the breasts is not achieved, particularly if the breasts are heavy.

- Discuss the need to check the position of the bra and prosthesis after raising the arms above the head.

- Discuss how to care for the prosthesis, i.e. washing and drying. Once the stuffing is dry it may require 'puffing up' to achieve its previous shape.

Many temporary breast forms allow the removal or addition of filling, so enabling the nurse to create a fuller or flatter form to meet more closely the needs of each woman. Sizes should only be used as a guideline.

It is advisable to secure the prosthesis within the bra using safety pins, press studs or stitches to prevent its moving and causing asymmetry and consequent embarrassment. Asymmetry may also occur when the arm on the affected side is raised, causing the bra to 'ride up' the chest wall and making realignment necessary. Such practical information may enable women to feel more secure and avoid embarrassing moments that could further damage their already reduced self-esteem.

Most women are able to wear a bra when they leave hospital, but some find it too uncomfortable and may prefer to have a temporary prosthesis fitted into a full length slip or camisole. A few choose not to wear a prosthesis at all, but must be given the opportunity to have one fitted.

Ideally, the fitting of the temporary prosthesis should be undertaken by an experienced ward nurse as part of routine post-operative care. The time taken to fit the prosthesis provides an ideal opportunity for the nurse to assess how the woman is coping with her surgery and her diagnosis of breast cancer. Discussion may include how she feels about looking at her scar and how her partner is responding. It is also a good time to discuss suitable bras and show her examples of permanent prostheses.

Women undergoing radiotherapy to the chest wall should wear a temporary prosthesis to avoid the pressure and irritation that might be caused by a heavier permanent breast prosthesis. There are several types of temporary or lighter breast prostheses.

PERMANENT BREAST PROSTHESES

Many different shapes and sizes of permanent breast prostheses are available today, manufactured by several companies (Appendix B). It should therefore be possible for all women to regain a symmetrical breast contour with a prosthesis following breast surgery.

Improved technology in recent years has meant that breast prostheses now resemble much more closely the size, shape, weight and feel of a breast when placed in the cup of a bra. Oil, foam, air, glass bead and seed fillings for prostheses have been replaced by those made of silicone gel. Most are slightly concave to allow close and comfortable contact with the chest wall, they will also retain the body's temperature so enhancing their natural feel.

There are four basic shapes of prostheses:

- asymmetrical with a tail of variable length to fill in any deficit of tissue under the arm;
- eliptical or oval;
- symmetrical;
- heart-shaped.

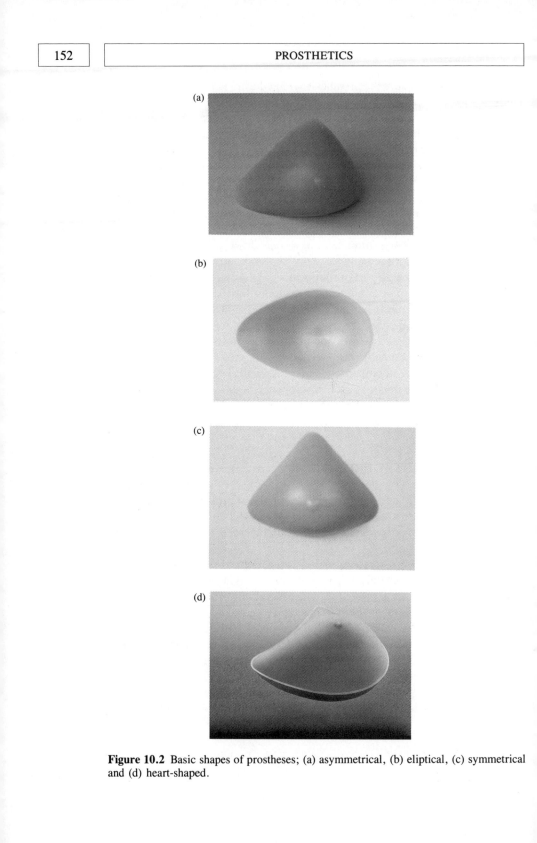

Figure 10.2 Basic shapes of prostheses; (a) asymmetrical, (b) eliptical, (c) symmetrical and (d) heart-shaped.

Examples of these are shown in Figure 10.2. Manufacturers make similar-shaped products but all are slightly different in a bra, so if a woman is to receive the best prosthesis for her she must have access to a wide range of products as well as a skilled and knowledgeable prosthetic fitter. Preferably this service should be provided in the hospital where she is being treated to maintain continuity of care.

Adaptations of the basic styles of prosthesis are available for women with heavy breasts or sensitive skins who may find a full prosthesis uncomfortable. Several companies manufacture 'light versions', which are hollowed out to reduce weight. Some very light prostheses are made by various manufacturers; they can be very useful for women with sensitive skins or persistent chest wall discomfort, but it is sometimes difficult to achieve such a close degree of symmetry with them because they are so much lighter than the remaining breast.

Women who cannot achieve a good result with these 'off the peg' prostheses may benefit from the 'made to measure' service offered by some companies. However, this process does take several weeks to complete and is far more expensive. For women who have had partial mastectomies, partial silicone prostheses are also available.

Unfortunately, manufacturers of breast prostheses in the UK continue to cater largely for a fair skinned population; there is inadequate provision for darker-skinned women. It is possible to colour a prosthesis for a woman if a material sample is provided matching her skin colour, but again this process takes several weeks and limits the woman's choice of prosthesis. Several shades of brown prostheses are routinely available in the USA and it is hoped that companies distributing in the UK will soon also provide a similar service. Currently only one company provides 'off the shelf' prosthetics in darker skin tones.

SILICONE NIPPLES

Most silicone breast prostheses have a nipple integral to their form. However, women with prominent nipples may wish to use separate silicone nipples, which can be affixed to the breast prosthesis using a little water or skin cream, to create a more even appearance in clothing. They are easily removed and re-applied as necessary. Many women find them particularly useful when wearing swimsuits, T-shirts or evening wear, and some women who have undergone breast reconstruction prefer to use silicone nipples to having nipple areolar complex reconstruction.

Silicone nipples are available from several manufacturers, but some hospitals make their own by taking a mould from the woman's remaining nipple. This is likely to produce the best result of all.

FITTING THE PERMANENT PROSTHESIS

At least 45 minutes should be allocated for each fitting for a silicone prosthesis to ensure it is not rushed and that a relaxed atmosphere is encouraged. If a nurse specialist is the fitter she may wish to allow longer so as to be able to assess the woman's physical and psychological well-being fully and discuss any problems being experienced.

The facilities for fitting prostheses should include a comfortable and private room with a full length mirror to allow the woman to observe her appearance with different prostheses. It is essential that the person fitting the prosthesis recognizes how vulnerable a woman may feel at this time, particularly if she has not met the prosthetic fitter before. She may feel embarrassed at revealing her scar to another person or apprehensive about the appearance of the prosthesis and the degree to which it will restore her natural shape. A sensitive approach by the fitter is important and is likely to increase the satisfaction a woman feels with the service given (Simpson, 1985).

A suitable bra

The success of a prosthetic fitting is, to a great extent, dependent on the type of bra a woman wears. Special mastectomy bras do exist and can be purchased from some specialist shops or companies, but prostheses will fit securely into many 'ordinary bras' that are supportive and fit correctly. Ideally, types of suitable bras should be discussd with a woman before she leaves hospital. Quite often she can continue to wear the bras she wore previously, but she may need to be re-measured and advised about styles and places to purchase suitable bras. An example of a suitable bra is given in Figure 10.3. Some hospitals stock a limited supply of bras or have samples of suitable styles. Ward nurses may find it helpful to build up a folder of information on suitable bras, local stockists and helpful local stores where staff have experience of dealing with women who have had breast surgery. Breast Cancer Care (fomerly the Breast Care and Mastectomy Association) will also provide information on underwear and clothing (Appendix A).

Modern prostheses are made to be worn in the bra cup next to the skin. However, a few women feel more secure if it is contained in a pocket attached to the bra. Some mastectomy bras already have pockets integral to their design, but pockets are easily added to other bras if a woman wishes. This can be undertaken by prosthetic companies, local agencies or the woman herself.

Choosing the correct prosthesis

After ensuring that the wound is well healed and that the woman has a suitable and correctly-fitting bra, the prosthesis can be chosen. The size and shape of the remaining breast should be observed within the bra, and the type and

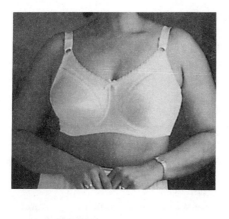

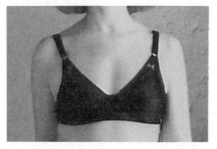

Figure 10.3 Suitable bras for women who have undergone a mastectomy. Photographs courtesy of CAMP Patient Care Group.

extent of surgery noted. This will allow the fitter to gauge which prostheses are most likely to be appropriate. Every woman should be given a choice of prostheses as the final decision will rest with her alone and will be based on comfort as well as appearance.

The woman should be shown how to place the prosthesis within the cup of the bra before observing herself in a mirror from the front and the side. It is helpful if she brings a tight fitting, light coloured, unpatterned T-shirt to wear with the prosthesis to allow a more critical appraisal of the shape created. She should also be encouraged to slide her hands over both breasts at the same time to ensure the shape of the prosthesis matches the distribution of breast tissue in her own breast. The fitter can check the distance between the centre of the bra and the nipple on both sides to ensure it is equal. A tape measure running from nipple to nipple should form a horizontal line; if it does not, the bra straps may need to be adjusted to correct it.

Following these guidelines most women will be able to obtain natural, equal breast contour with a silicone prosthesis. However, some women, who seemed happy with the chosen prosthesis initially may find they are not happy after wearing it for a length of time. They should be encouraged to return and discuss any problems with the fitter. They should also be aware of how to look after the prosthesis and their entitlement to new prostheses in the future. These are summarized in Table 3.

INFORMATION FOR WOMEN USING A SILICONE BREAST PROSTHESIS

A silicone prosthesis is made to be worn next to the skin, but a soft cover is also supplied with each prosthesis to be worn as desired. This may be more comfortable in hot weather.

Prostheses should be washed daily with warm water and soap, and dried using a towel. They should not be placed on anything hot, such as a radiator, and talcum powder, creams or oils should not be applied directly to their surface.

All prostheses have a one year guarantee at least but with careful handling will usually last for two to three years. All NHS patients are entitled to breast prostheses free of charge. Private patients must purchase prostheses, but most health insurance companies will cover at least the cost of the first prosthesis obtained.

A woman is entitled to a new prosthesis if she loses weight, her breasts change shape or when the prosthesis shows signs of wear, e.g. bubbles appear, it cracks or loses shape.

Silicone prostheses are very hardy but will split if pierced with a sharp implement, so care should be taken when wearing brooches or handling pets. If it splits, sticky silicone will be exposed, but covering the split with tape will allow time to obtain a replacement prosthesis.

A silicone prosthesis is impervious to salt water or chlorine and can safely be used when swimming, although it should always be worn within a pocket in the swimsuit to prevent it moving or falling out.

Special mastectomy bras and swimsuits do exist but tend to be more expensive. Many ordinary bras and swimsuits can be adapted to accommodate a silicone prosthesis securely. Underwired garments are not generally advised as they are likely to damage the prosthesis.

Strapless bras can still be worn but some women find a silicone prosthesis too heavy to wear in them and so use a lighter or temporary prosthesis when wearing a strapless bra.

Most clothing can continue to be worn following a mastectomy and the use of a silicone prosthesis. Low-cut garments can frequently be adapted using lace, elastic or ornamental additions to enable a woman to feel secure and confident.

If women experience problems with their prosthesis or are not happy with it they should contact their breast care nurse or prosthetic fitter. Breast Cancer Care also provides information on the types and availability of breast prostheses and practical information on bras and clothing.

CLOTHING ADVICE

Many women are concerned that they will be unable to wear fashionable, feminine styles of clothing, particularly evening wear and swimsuits following a mastectomy. This is not so. Strapless, low-back or off-the-shoulder dresses are all still possible. No clothes should automatically be discarded. Plunging necklines may no longer be appropriate, but many such clothes can be adapted using contrasting materials, lace or jewellery to create a different but equally pleasing effect.

When wearing a strapless bra, a light, soft, temporary prosthesis may be preferred to the heavier silicone type. However, there are now prosthetics that may be worn with adhesives to stick them to the chest wall so giving more security when wearing a strapless bra. Some women with smaller prostheses may be able to go without a bra for short periods of time. This type of prosthesis is available from several prosthetic companies.

SWIMSUITS

The styles of swimwear that can be worn will depend on the type of surgery performed and the position of the scar. Specially made mastectomy costumes are available from certain shops and some companies offer a mail order service. The range is becoming greater and more interesting but they tend to be more expensive than 'normal' swimwear.

Many high street stores now sell swimsuits that are suitable for women who have had mastectomies. Some may require small adjustments in order to ensure that the prosthesis can be securely held in place and that the scar is not visible. Bikinis can also be worn very successfully, particularly the bandeau style. When wearing any swimsuit, the silicone prosthesis must be secured within a pocket to prevent it moving or falling out. Some women prefer to use a temporary or foam prosthesis in costumes but should remember to squeeze it discreetly after leaving the water to prevent water being retained by the prosthesis and its becoming visible.

The Breast Cancer Care Association provides very useful information about clothing and swimwear as well as bras and prostheses.

REFERENCES

Denton, S. and Baum, M. (1983) Psychological aspects of Breast Cancer in *Breast Cancer* (ed. R. Margolese), Churchill Livingstone, Edinburgh.

Maguire, P., Lee, E.G., Bevington, D.J. *et al.* (1978) Psychiatric problems in the first year after mastectomy. *British Medical Journal* 15 April, 963–5.

Simpson, G. (1985) Are you being served? *Senior Nurse* 2(6) 14–16.

Diet and breast cancer | 11

Maureen Hunter and Clare Shaw

DIET IN THE AETIOLOGY OF BREAST CANCER

There is an increasing amount of evidence to suggest that diet may play a role in the aetiology of cancer and it is estimated that an average of 35% of all cancers may be attributable to diet (Bingham, 1990). The possible association between diet and breast cancer has been the subject of particular attention, interest and research. Early experiments showed that high fat diets were an effective means of promoting tumour growth in animals with chemically-induced mammary tumours. Total energy intake also appeared to influence tumour growth, with high energy intakes causing tumour promotion. The effects of fat and energy intakes appear to be separate (Schatzkin *et al.*, 1989).

Interest in the role played by dietary fat in humans originated in epidemiological studies, particularly correlation studies. There is a 5.5-fold range in breast cancer incidence throughout the world and dietary fat consumption also shows a wide range. When analysed, the two tend to show a strong positive correlation (Rose, 1986). This association is present for both pre-and post-menopausal women, although it is stronger for the latter.

The advantage of such studies is that a wide range of both fat intake and breast cancer rates can be examined. Comparison of fat intake between countries provides a greater range of intakes than would be seen between individuals in any one country. One drawback, however, is that the data used for per capita fat consumption is derived from figures relating to the availability of fat and tends to be an overestimate of individual consumption. This may be particularly true of Western countries where food wastage may be high.

Some countries do not fit in to the correlation particularly well. Israel shows a disproportionately higher rate of breast cancer than would be expected from per capita fat intake (Hirayama, 1978). This may be explained in part by the great variation in the incidence of breast cancer among various ethnic groups in the country, with those of European origin having higher rates than those from Asia and Africa.

Studies of migrant populations have helped to examine the possibility that genetic differences may account for some of the world-wide variation in breast cancer rates. Women migrating from an area of low incidence to one of high incidence have a tendency to have acquired a similar rate of breast cancer to that of their host country by the second generation. This has been observed in successive generations of Japanese women who migrated to Hawaii (Willet, 1990). Gradual dietary changes to a higher fat intake may be a major influence. Although there is a tendency for breast cancer to run in families, which points to a genetic influence, these studies illustrate that environmental factors can dramatically alter the incidence of breast cancer in a population group over time.

Changes in the diet of populations have also provided supporting evidence for a link between environmental factors and breast cancer. Dietary changes have occurred in Japan over the past 40 years: per capita daily fat intake rose from 23 g per day to 52 g per day between 1957/59 and 1973. Breast cancer rates also rose over this period, by approximately 30% (Hirayama, 1978). Similar changes have been seen in other countries such as Iceland. Urban areas in countries such as Japan tend to adopt Western-style diets much more rapidly than rural areas. Breast cancer rates for Japanese women tend to be higher in cities and in women of higher socio-economic groups (Rose, 1986).

Although correlation studies can provide indications of dietary links with disease, it is thought that more conclusive evidence is obtained from case control and cohort studies. Case control studies compare the previous dietary habits of breast cancer patients with those of non-cancer patients. Such research has shown only weak positive associations, or no association, between dietary fat intake and breast cancer. When controlling for the effect of particular nutrients, the relative risk rose with increasing consumption of beef, red meats, pork and sweet desserts (Boyle and Leake, 1988).

Poor correlations may arise because of problems inherent in the methodology. Dietary fat intake varies within a limited range in a given population so that little difference may be observed in the mean intake of cases and controls. The lower end of the range may still be too high to influence breast cancer risk. Assessment of intake by questionnaire produces additional errors because of the difficulty of determining accurate food intake. The dietary intake of cancer patients may change once a diagnosis has been made as individuals become more aware of their health.

Cohort studies record the current intakes of healthy individuals who are then followed up. The diets of individuals who develop cancer is then compared with those who remain healthy. An advantage is that diagnosis or illness does not influence the dietary intake as this is recorded prior to the disease. In addition, information can be obtained about diet over a period of time before diagnosis. Large numbers are needed for cohort studies and follow-up over a considerable time period is required. The results of cohort studies have shown mildly positive correlations, no association and even weak negative associations between dietary fat and breast cancer (Schatzkin et al., 1989).

The most reliable evidence for dietary fat influence in the development of breast cancer originates from intervention studies. A number of researchers have undertaken feasibility studies on the use of low fat diets in women with breast cancer or those at increased risk of the disease (Boyar et al., 1988). Dietary intervention has generally been aimed at reducing fat intake so that people are gaining 20% of their energy from fat compared with the average of approximately 40% in many Western countries. Women need to undergo dietary counselling from a dietitian with regular follow-up to achieve such a change in their diet. Current dietary guidelines for the general population recommend a reduction of fat to 30% of total energy intake in the long term (NACNE, 1983). Very low fat diets are difficult to follow, particularly when dining out or catering for a family. Women need to be highly motivated and have an incentive if they are to follow such a diet for an extended period of time. Some dietary intervention studies are currently being carried out. They have identified that women are able to adhere to a sufficiently low fat diet (Boyd et al., 1992; Boyar et al., 1988) but as yet have failed to show a reduction in the rate of breast cancer.

Some dietary intervention studies are currently being carried out. One large scale trial, 'the Women's Health Trial' was planned to take place in the USA. It aimed to reduce the fat intake of middle-aged women to determine if breast cancer incidence would be reduced. Discussions led to the trial being suspended as the numbers and period of follow-up required exceeded available funding. However, it has been emphasized that important evidence is unlikely to arise from any source other than such intervention studies (Prentice et al., 1988).

Since the mid-1960's there has been a suggestion that obesity increases the risk of breast cancer in post-menopausal women (de Ward, Baanders-van Halewijn and Huizinga, 1964). A number of studies have since come to the same conclusion (Kelsey et al., 1981; Lubin et al., 1985) although some have suggested that the effect of being overweight or obese proved to be small (de Waard, 1993). An important factor may be the age since menopause, as the positive relationship between body weight and age appears stronger for women who are five years or more beyond the menopause (Rose, 1986). It has been suggested that obese women with breast cancer are more likely to develop metastases and have a shorter survival time (Rose, 1990; Senie et al., 1992). Intervention studies have failed to show an improved survival with weight reduction in obese post menopausal women (de Waard et al., 1993). This may be explained in part by the introduction of tamoxifen during the course of the study, which had a profound effect on prognosis.

The risks associated with body weight appear to be the opposite for pre-menopausal women, with thin pre-menopausal women being at increased risk (Rose et al., 1986). Possible mechanisms for the link between obesity and breast cancer have been proposed and oestrogen is particularly implicated. Circulating oestrogens, especially non-bound oestrogen, have an important stimulatory effect on the growth of mammary tissue. The effect may be synergistic with prolactin and regulated at a cellular level by other growth factors. Obesity is thought to raise oestrogen levels by increasing the conversion of oestrone to oestradiol from its adrenal precursor androsesteredione, in adipose tissue (Ingram et al., 1989). Aromatase enzymes are responsible for this conversion.

The elevation of plasma oestrogens by an increase in fat cell production and the possibility that dietary fat may influence ovarian hormonal production directly are two simplistic links proposed for the connection between dietary fat and breast cancer. A very low fat diet is capable of reducing plasma oestradiol after a period of five months (Boyar et al., 1988), and citizens of countries where a low fat diet is habitually consumed have lower plasma oestrogens. However, elevated plasma oestrogens are not generally reported from studies of breast cancer patients.

The influence that dietary fat and oestrogens have is likely to occur over a number of years. It is known that early menarche, late menopause and nulliparity are associated with increased risk. All these factors involve an increased exposure to oestrogens and a reduced lifetime exposure to prolactin compared with women who experience a late menarche, early menopause and early first pregnancy. Overnutrition and a high fat diet may exacerbate such exposure.

Other ideas that have been proposed include an effect of dietary fat on membrane permeability, prostaglandin synthesis, immune function, DNA repair and metabolism of chemical carcinogens (Schatzkin et al., 1989). Although a link appears possible, the mechanism of action still requires further investigation.

Other nutrients have been implicated as having a potential role in the development of breast cancer. Dietary fibre is known to influence oestrogen metabolism via the enterohepatic circulation. Vegetarians consuming a diet high in dietary fibre have been shown to have higher faecal oestrogen excretion. Plasma oestrogens were negatively correlated with faecal excretion, and it has also been shown that fibre supplementation has the potential to reduce plasma oestrone (Rose and Connolly, 1990). The magnitude of effect and the overall implications are, as yet, unclear.

Alcohol has also been identified as having a possible association with the development of breast cancer. A review by Hiatt (1990) shows that 10 out of 16 case control studies and five out of six cohort studies have produced results supporting a positive association. Risk seems to rise with an average consumption of one to two drinks daily, although there is little agreement as to whether a dose–response relationship exists. There is, as yet, no known biological mechanism by which alcohol consumption leads to cancer of the breast. It has been suggested (Harvey et al., 1987) that the influence on hepatic enzymes, inhibition of hepatic oestrogen metabolism or stimulation of prolactin from the pituitary may be possible modes of action. Data available at present is far from conclusive that alcohol is a contributory causal factor in breast cancer development. Further studies are required before specific dietary guidelines can be issued.

Evidence so far, although not conclusive, points towards the idea that dietary intervention may have a role to play in breast cancer prevention and in influencing prognosis. Maintenance of ideal body weight and modification of dietary fat, dietary fibre and possibly alcohol appear to be the most likely dietary factors to influence breast cancer development. Further research is required before definite quantitative or qualitative guidelines can be made.

HORMONAL THERAPIES AND OBESITY

Treatment for breast cancer may involve endocrine intervention such as the use of tamoxifen. Tamoxifen is now regarded as an effective means of delaying relapse and prolonging survival in women with primary breast cancer (Medical Research Council Scottish Trials Office, 1987). Weight gain is now recognized as a potential side-effect of tamoxifen therapy. Not all studies have agreed with this finding, however, and not all women will necessarily increase their body weight (Powles et al., 1989).

Oral megestrol acetate and medroxyprogesterone acetate are also used in the treatment of breast cancer. Their action is different to that of tamoxifen although the reported response rate is similar (Sedlacek, 1988). Both may be used on women who have previously relapsed on other endocrine manipulations. Megestrol acetate has a greater capacity to promote appetite and weight gain. It may be helpful to warn women about the potential for weight gain and to suggest they seek appropriate advice from a dietitian. In advanced disease megestrol acetate or medroxyprogesterone acetate may provide a useful pharmaceutical intervention in women with cancer cachexia due to its capacity to stimulate appetite and promote weight gain.

DIET AND LYMPHOEDEMA

From as early as 1948 obesity has been cited as a contributory risk factor for the development of lymphoedema (MacDonald, 1948). Of a series of women undergoing surgery from 1966, 85% weighed more than 80kg (Clodius, 1977). Other studies that have looked at obesity as a risk factor for lymphoedema have tended to examine the absolute weight of patients who have developed lymphoedema. Such studies do not take into account the degree of obesity or body mass index prior to the development of the swelling (Treves, 1957). Some researchers have reported a therapeutic use of low fat diets in the treatment of lymphoedema (Mirabile *et al.*, 1991). Further research is required to determine the role of obesity as a risk factor for the development of lymphoedema and whether dietary intervention can aid its treatment.

THE NUTRITIONAL CARE OF WOMEN WITH BREAST CANCER

The aims of nutritional care in patients with cancer are:

- to maintain optimal nutritional status;
- to overcome eating difficulties that may arise as a result of the disease or treatment and to enable patients to enjoy their food and thus have an enhanced quality of life.

Once a woman has been diagnosed as having breast cancer it is important for her to maintain a good nutritional status before, during and after her course of treatment. A reduction in nutritional status leads to weight loss and malnutrition, which in turn leads to muscle wasting, a depressed immune response, impaired wound healing, electrolyte and fluid imbalances, low morale and progressive weakness. This may then compromise the patient's tolerance of, and response to, anticancer therapy (Shils, 1979).

If a woman is already showing signs of malnutrition on diagnosis, every effort should be made to restore status before treatment is begun. The nutritional care of women with breast cancer can be divided into two areas:

1. women who present at diagnosis or for treatment with an optimum nutritional status;
2. women who present with a poor nutritional status, or whose nutritional status begins to deteriorate during the course of treatment or as disease progresses.

Nutritional care of women with optimum nutritional status

When newly diagnosed as having breast cancer, most women present without any nutritional difficulties. They are often very interested in general nutrition and the concept of maintaining a healthy, well-balanced diet. Women in this category should be given general healthy eating advice.

The concept of healthy eating involves taking a well-balanced diet that provides all the energy, protein, vitamins, minerals and fibre that the body requires, and also avoiding an excessive intake of fat, sugar, commercial or manufactured foods and salt. In addition to the links between diet and cancer, it is known that diet can influence the development of other diseases, particularly obesity, hypertension, heart disease and bowel disorders. The important recommended guidelines for healthy eating are listed below.

Reducing dietary fat

The majority of fat intake comes from meat products. However, this does not mean that a vegetarian diet will be low in fat, as the next highest sources of fat are milk, cooking oils, butter, cakes and pastries, cheese, cream and eggs. Some of the dietary fat eaten comes from saturated fats, which are mainly of animal origin; polyunsaturated fats come from vegetable sources. While saturated fats are thought to be the most detrimental in terms of raising cholesterol, the advice is to reduce the total fat intake.

Increasing dietary fibre

Most dietary fibre comes from vegetables, then cereals and breads, and then fruit. An increase in consumption of these fibre-rich foods also means an increased intake of the vitamins and minerals contained in them, for example, vitamin C and vitamin A.

Reducing dietary sugar

As well as being added to foods and drinks by individuals, sugar is eaten in processed foods such as cakes, sweets, chocolates, fizzy drinks and even some sauces and soups. Reducing consumption of these foods as well as reducing added sugar, will help to reduce total dietary sugar.

Women presenting at diagnosis or for treatment may be overweight. It may be appropriate for them to lose it, but this is a decision that must only be made after consultation with the patient's doctor. The patient should then be referred to a dietitian for weight-reducing advice.

Nutritional care of women with poor nutritional status

A reduction in nutritional status arises from a prolonged period of poor food intake and from metabolic alterations caused by the disease state itself. A reduction in food intake may result from the presence of the disease or its treatment.

Factors that can cause a reduction in food intake in women with breast cancer include:

- anxiety;
- depression;
- side-effects of chemotherapy such as anorexia, nausea and vomiting;
- side-effects of radiotherapy, such as anorexia and nausea.

The abnormalities of metabolism that occur in cancer patients include an alteration in the metabolism of glucose in cancer cells. This leads to an increase in the energy requirements of the cancer patient (von Meyenfeldt *et al.*, 1988).

Table 11.1 Common eating difficulties and remedies

Eating difficulty	Possible cause	Guidelines for dietary suggestions
Appetite loss	Systemic and metabolic effects of disease	Small portions of nourishing meals with snacks and/or nourising drinks in between. Nutritional supplements may be useful.
Severe appetite loss	Systemic and metabolic effects of disease	Appetite stimulants such as alcohol or prednisolone may be helpful. Supplementary nasogastric feeding may be appropriate if problem persists.
Nausea	Chemotherapy	As above and try: avoiding unpleasant odours or smells and very sweet or very fatty foods; choosing cold foods (these have less smell), fizzy drinks, dry meals with drinks taken half an hour before or after, fresh air before meals.
Severe nausea and/or vomiting	Chemotherapy	As above. Total Parenteral Nutrition may be appropriate if problem persists. NB It is assumed that appropriate anti emetic cover is given.
Taste changes	Chemotherapy	Avoid foods known to accentuate unpleasant taste. Enhance food flavour by using sauces, condiments and marinades, etc.
Weight loss	Metabolic effect of disease, prolonged poor food intake	Increase food intake by modifying diet to reduce problem causing poor food intake. Little and often. Appropriate use of nutritional supplements.

If they are not met, the patient is at risk of weight loss and deterioration in nutritional status. To avoid this, women should be referred to a dietitian for assessment and advice as soon as nutritional status begins to deteriorate. Indications of this might be:

- when the patient has lost 10% or more of her normal weight;
- when weight loss is progressive, although perhaps not more than 10%;
- when the presence of any eating difficulties continues to limit the patient's food intake.

Nutritional support in these women usually takes the form of normal diet, or modifications of a normal diet, with the use of nutritional supplements. Some common eating difficulties and suggested ways of helping to overcome them are shown in Table 11.1.

Nutritional supplements

There are many nutritional support products now available that are very useful in the nutritional care of patients. All must be used only in conjunction with dietary advice and under the supervision of a dietitian.

Commercially available nourishing drinks

It is possible to make home-made nourishing drinks from everyday ingredients such as milk, ice-cream, cream and so on. However, there are specially formulated drinks available that are useful as meal replacements or as supplementary drinks taken in between meals. Some are powders that are reconstituted with milk, such as Build Up (Nestlé), or water such as Complan (Glaxo). Ready to use nourishing drinks are also available, such as Fresubin (Fresenius), Liquisorb (Merck), Ensure Plus (Abbott) and Fortisip (Cow & Gate). All come in a wide range of flavours, both sweet and savoury. Most are available on prescription (with the exception of Build Up and Complan).

Commercially available energy and protein supplements

These are available as powders or liquids that can be added to food or drinks and are a useful way of increasing energy and protein intake as appropriate.

Energy supplements Glucose polymer powders are white tasteless powders that look like glucose. They can be added to drinks and used in recipes to increase the energy content without altering the taste. Examples include: Maxijul (Scientific Hospital Supplies), Polycose (Abbott) and Polycal (Cow & Gate).

Glucose drinks are also available. These come in a variety of flavours and can be mixed with lemonades, fizzy drinks, fruit juices or milk shakes. They can also be used in jellies, puddings and ice lollies. Examples include: Polycal (Cow & Gate), Hycal (Smith Kline Beecham) and Maxijul (Scientific Hospital Supplies).

Protein supplements These are powdered protein supplements that can be added to drinks or foods such as milky drinks, puddings or soups. Examples include: Maxipro HBV Super Soluble (Scientific Hospital Supplies), Casilan (Crookes) and Protifar (Cow & Gate). New supplements appear regularly. Ask a dietitian for the latest information.

COMPLEMENTARY AND ALTERNATIVE DIETARY THERAPIES

These are unusual modificiations to a normal diet which are claimed to benefit patients with cancer. They are normally recommended in conjunction with (complementary) or instead of (alternative) conventional anticancer treatments. Most originate from the Far East or the USA and they are popular with cancer patients, particularly women with breast cancer.

The diets are not generally isolated regimes but are part of a programme of activities aimed at increasing patients' well-being that includes such things as relaxation, therapeutic massage and so on.

A number of these diets are currently popular with differing degrees of dietary restrictions. Some claim to cure, while others claim to benefit the patient by increasing well-being, reducing symptoms and promoting a positive attitude.

The diets share similar dietary guidelines. They are generally low in fat, high in fibre, low in salt, low in sugar and mostly strict vegetarian or vegan regimes. Some of the programmes also recommend megadose vitamin therapy, such as large doses of vitamins A and C, and make other unusual recommendations, such as the taking of pancreatic enzymes or coffee enemas.

The benefit of these diets seems to be associated with the positive attitude and feeling of control that they impart, which patients are often seeking. It is unlikely that the diets alone offer any real medical benefit that results from their nutrient content. In fact, these diets often prove harmful, especially if followed to the exclusion of conventional treatment. This is because the severity of them may result in a reduced total energy intake, which leads to weight loss and a deterioration in nutritional status. Many patients choose to follow such regimes when they may already be experiencing eating difficulties and weight loss. Eating a diet high in bulk is very difficult in the presence of eating difficulties and this, combined with the low energy content, may further reduce nutritional status.

For these reasons, women following or contemplating following such regimes should be referred to a dietitian for advice. It is sometimes possible to accommodate certain aspects of these diets into a properly planned nutritional programme providing that they do not have harmful effects or interfere with treatment.

Like all complementary therapies, it is a matter of individual choice for the woman herself. However, she must be given sufficient, balanced information about the advantages and disadvantages of such dietary therapies to be able to make an informed choice. Any woman choosing to follow one of these regimes must have her nutritional status assessed and monitored regularly by a dietitian to ensure that the woman is not placing herself nutritionally at risk. It should be stressed to patients that the most important point about any diet, whether 'normal' or 'complementary', is that it should provide a good, well-balanced food intake so as to achieve or maintain optimum nutritional status.

REFERENCES

Bingham, S. (1990) *Diet and Cancer Briefing Paper*, Health Education Authority and Department of Health, London.

Boyar, A.P., Rose, D.P., Loughridge, J.R. *et al.* (1988) Response to a diet low in total fat in women with postmenopausal breast cancer: a pilot study. *Nutr. Cancer*, **11**(2), 93–9.

Boyd, N.F., Cousins, M., Lockwood, G. and Tritchler, D. (1990) The feasibility of testing experimentally the dietary fat–breast cancer hypothesis. *Prog. Clin. Biol. Res.*, **346**, 231–41.

Boyle, P. and Leake, R. (1988) Progress in understanding breast cancer: epidemiology and biological interactions. *Breast Cancer Research and Treatment*, **11**, 91–112.

Clodius, L. (1977) Secondary Arm Lymphoedema, in (1977) *Lymphoedema* (ed. L. Clodius), Thienne, Stuttgart, p. 151.

de Waard, F., Baanders-van Halewijn, E.A. and Huizinga, J. (1964) The bimodal age distribution of patients with mammary carcinoma. *Cancer*, **17**, 141–51.

de Waard, E., Ramlau, R., Mulders, Y. *et al.* (1993) A feasibility study on weight reduction in obese postmenopausal breast cancer patients. *Eur. J. of Cancer Prev.*, **2**, 233–8.

Harvey, E.B., Schairer, C., Brinton, L.A. *et al.* (1987) Alcohol consumption and breast cancer. *Journal of the National Cancer Institute*, **28**(4), 657–61.

Hiatt, R.A. (1990) Alcohol consumption and breast cancer. *Medical Oncology and Tumour Pharmacotherapy*, **7**(213), 143–51.

Hirayama, T. (1978) Epidemiology of breast cancer with special reference to the role of diet. *Preventative Medicine*, **7**, 173–95.

Ingram, D., Nottage, E. Ng, S. *et al.* (1989) Obesity and breast disease, the role of female sex hormones. *Cancer*, **64**, 1049–53.

Kelsey, J.L., Fischer, D.B., Holford, T.R. *et al.* (1981) Exogenous oestrogens and other factors in epidemiology of breast cancer. *NHCI*, **67**, 327–33.

Lubin, F., Ruder, A.M., Wax, Y. and Modan, B. (1985) Overweight and changes in weight throughout adult life in breast cancer aetiology. *Am. J. Epid.*, **122**, 579–88.

MacDonald, I. (1948) Resection of the axillary vein in radical mastectomy: its relation to the mechanism of lymphoedema. *Cancer*, November, 618–22.

Medical Research Council Scottish Trials Office (1987) Adjuvant tamoxifen in the management of operable breast cancer; the Scottish trial. *Lancet*, 25 July, 171–5.

Mirabile, V., Placucci, P., Mazzoleni, C. *et al.* (1992) Preliminary results of diet-therapy. *Progress in Lymphology*, **XIII**, 559–60, Ed. R.V. Cluzan, A.P. Pecking, F.M. Lokiec, Pub. Excerpta Medica, London.

National Advisory Committee on Nutrition Education (1983) *Proposals for Nutritional Guidelines for Health Education in Britain*, Health Education Council, London.

Powles, T.J., Hardy, J.R., Ashley, S.E. *et al.* (1989) A pilot trial to evaluate the acute toxicity and feasibility of tamoxifen for prevention of breast cancer. *British Journal of Cancer*, **60**, 126–31.

Prentice, R.L., Kakar, F., Hursting, S. *et al.* (1988) Aspects for the rationale for the Women's Health Trial. *Journal of the National Cancer Institute*, **80**(11), 802–14.

Rose, D.P. (1986) Dietary factors and breast cancer. *Cancer Surveys*, **5**(3), 671–87.

Rose, D.P. and Connolly, J.M. (1990) Dietary prevention of breast cancer. *Med. Oncology and Tumour Pharmacotherapy*, **7**, 121–30.

Schatzkin, A., Greenwald, P., Byar, D.P. and Clifford, C.K. (1989) The dietary fat–breast cancer hypothesis is alive. *Journal of the American Medical Association*, **261**(22), 3284–7.

Sedlacek, S.M. (1988) An overview of megestrol acetate for the treatment of advanced breast cancer. *Seminars in Oncology*, **15**, 2nd supplement, 3–13.

Senie, R.T., Rosen, P.P., Rhodes, P. *et al.* (1992) obesity at diagnosis of breast carcinoma influences duration of disease free survival. *Annals of Internal Medicine*, **116**, 26–32.

Shils, M. (1979) Principles of nutritional therapy. *Cancer*, **43**, 2093–2102.

Treves, N. (1957) An evaluation of etiological factors of lymphedema following radical mastectomy. *Cancer*, **10**, 444–59.

von Meyenfeldt, M.F., Fredix, E.W.H.M., Haagh, W.A.J.J.M. *et al.* (1988) The aetiology and management of weight loss and malnutrition in cancer patients. *Baillière's Clinical Gastroenterology*, Volume 2, Part 4, 869–85, Baillière Tindall, London.

The nursing management of malignant fungating breast lesions

12

Kate Gowshall

The care of patients with malignant fungating breast lesions poses an enormous challenge for nurses and the problem faced by the patients is often extreme. Doyle (1980) graphically describes what these patients may experience:

> Can we begin to imagine what it must feel like for a patient to see part of his/her body rotting and to have to live with the offensive smell from it, see the reaction of his visitors (including doctors and nurses) and to know that it signifies lingering death?

The way nurses approach this problem significantly affects the quality of care given. Individual assessment of psychological, physical, emotional and spiritual needs is essential for the maintenance and promotion of the optimum quality of life for these patients. Awareness of and sensitivity to the psychological problems that a patient with a malignant fungating lesion may be experiencing is equally as important as control of the physical symptoms (Bennett, 1985).

THE NATURE OF FUNGATING LESIONS

Breast cancer is the commonest neoplasm to fungate. Malignant fungating lesions develop as a result of cancerous infiltration of the epithelium, lymph nodes and blood vessels, particularly capillaries (Foltz, 1980; Sims and Fitzgerald, 1985). This develops, leading to skin breakdown and thus to an ulcerating fungating mass (Figure 12.1). Local infection, malodour, excess exudate and bleeding may subsequently occur.

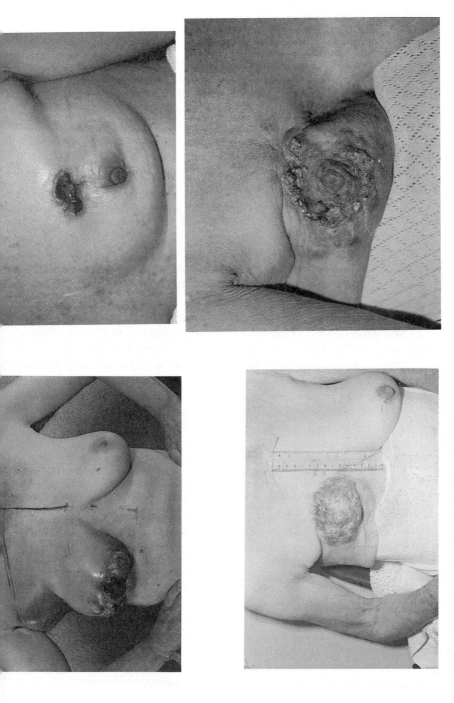

Figure 12.1 Examples of malignant fungating lesions.

The diagnosis of malignant fungating lesions still occasionally causes confusion. Rosen (1980) argues that they can be mistaken for benign dermal or subcutaneous growths. Although diagnosis is usually obvious, histological confirmation is required before treatment. This can be achieved easily in the majority of cases by Trucut needle biopsy under local anaesthesia.

A poor medical prognosis is often associated with this type of breast lesion. Petrek, Glenn and Craner (1983) consider patients incurable if presenting with skin ulceration of the breast, even in the absence of metastatic disease. However, Ivelic and Lyne (1990) cite Bloom, Richards and Harris (1962) who found that patients survived for many years following presentation of a malignant fungating mass.

Confusion surrounds the incidence and progression of fungating breast lesions and there is a paucity of published work on the condition. In a study of records from a London hospital, Bloom, Richards and Harris (1962) discovered that between 1880 and 1930 68% of women with breast cancer had some degree of ulceration. Haagensen (1971) reports that 5% of women with breast cancer present with ulceration, but this figure does not include women who go on to develop ulceration following progression of the disease. Thomas (1992) estimated the incidence of fungating lesions by surveying radiotherapy centres, hospices and specialist nurses and suggests that fungating lesions occur in sufficient number to represent a significant problem.

The overall number of patients with malignant fungating breast cancer is difficult to assess accurately because of poor documentation. It is possible that nurses consider malignant fungating breast lesions to be more prevalent than they actually are because they remember each case so vividly. Over recent years, advances in treatments and diagnostic techniques, as well as an increase in public awareness and health education, have contributed to a reduction in the number of malignant fungating breast lesions seen, although locally advanced breast disease is still too common (Kumar *et al.*, 1987).

The presentation of malignant fungating lesions falls into three categories.

1. Rapidly progressive breast cancers (usually inflammatory in nature). These cancers are often insensitive to many treatments.
2. Local recurrent breast cancer, seen after initial diagnosis/treatment.
3. Women who fail to seek advice for many years and present with an ulcerating/fungating lesion.

Women in the first two categories have often tried many different treatments for their recurrent fungating breast lesions and yet have experienced a return of the cancer, which has continued to fungate. These women often feel completely despondent, and despair of the problem ever being controlled. They may also feel angry with the disease and the failure of treatments, and have many fears about the future. They form a very different group to women in category 3 who seek help very late. Far too many women still fall into this latter group, and their reasons for failing to seek advice earlier are varied.

- Women may be afraid to seek advice because they fear:
- a diagnosis of cancer
- the consequences of diagnosis
- the unknown
- death.
- Women may be afraid to seek advice because they fear:
- an altered body image
- the loss of a breast
- the loss of sexuality
- a change or disruption in lifestyle
- for the future.
- These women may also feel:
- embarrassed
- self-conscious
- unclean
- a loss of self-respect
- guilty
- a sense of denial.
- They may not have sought advice from a specialist because:
- of other commitments, i.e. caring for an elderly or sick relative
- they had previously been dissatisfied or turned away by a GP.

The sensitivity of the nurses caring for these women is most important. The approach must be non-judgemental. The individual's problems should be identified and gently addressed, to increase self-confidence and allow for discussions and decisions on treatment options. Above all, respect for the patient and any previous decision not to seek help is important. They need positive reassurance, encouragement and counselling.

Patients who have not previously had treatment for their breast cancer may be extremely frightened and feel both vulnerable and guilty that they have not previously sought help, or they might now regret having asked for it. Their tumours do often respond to treatment and control can frequently be achieved.

PRESENTATION OF FUNGATING LESIONS

The fungating breast lesion presents as a primary cancer or as a recurrent breast cancer.

Early signs of fungating lesions

The woman's skin often becomes red, shiny, dry and very itchy. Eczema-like areas of unhealing broken skin develop and begin to discharge. Women may find this extremely frightening.

Three types of recurrence commonly occur following mastectomy or lumpectomy (Blackley, 1986).

1. Spot recurrence – a discrete circumspect nodule of malignant cells.
2. Multiple spot recurrences scattered over the scar.
3. Involvement of the whole area of skin with a moist thickened eczematous appearance.

These can lead to later problems and will ulcerate/fungate if they are not treated or if treatment fails.

The red, dry appearance of the skin may gradually spread across the entire chest. The skin is very friable and needs to be treated with great care. Those affected often complain of tightness and itchiness which is painful and extremely uncomfortable. It is usually preferable for nothing to be applied to the skin because of its fragility; it is hoped that the tumour will respond to medical treatments. The itchiness causes great concern and breakdown of the skin is often accelerated if it is scratched.

Antihistamines can be prescribed, but many women are reluctant to take them because of the side-effect of drowsiness; occasionally women find herbal remedies of some use. Analgesics are also very important as the area can be painful. The discharging areas are usually covered, but it is important to avoid the use of too much tape on the friable skin. Advice on soft support cotton bras is necessary to promote comfort.

Psychological problems can be enormous. Actually to witness the cancer spreading causes great trauma and fear, and women often become very distressed, anxious and depressed. Endocrine therapy is sometimes the treatment of choice and it is usually some six weeks before any obvious response can be seen; when a woman is living with and seeing this locally recurrent disease, six weeks can seem an unbearably long time. Affected women often feel very limited with clothing and feel they need to hide this angry red skin that represents their breast cancer and the threat to their life.

Later signs of fungating lesions

The skin area continues to be very friable, the discharge increases and the area becomes ulcerated and fails to heal. Infection often sets in and the area then becomes malodorous. Bleeding – slight, moderate or severe – can arise, and the whole area can be very painful. The nursing management is discussed later.

THE AIMS OF TREATMENT

Treatment of a fungating breast lesion is not intended to be curative. The aim is to control and palliate: controlling symptoms and promoting optimum quality of life. The methods used are:

- chemotherapy
- endocrine therapy
- radiotherapy
- palliative surgery
- symptom control.

The pathological basis of the fungating lesion – the cancer – must be treated. If the cancer does not respond, healing and regression of the fungating lesion will not occur.

Chemotherapy is often used for rapidly progressing lesions or to reduce tumour bulk to allow for a surgical procedure. The effects of chemotherapy can be very debilitating.

Endocrine therapy is often used for more slowly progressing lesions, and also as first line treatment for women who have failed to seek early advice. Endocrine therapies are slow to take effect and frustration and despondency may occur.

Radiotherapy is often used to reduce tumour bulk, either to improve management or prior to surgical procedures. It is occasionally used to control bleeding.

Palliative surgery is occasionally indicated for the control of fungating lesions, often after a course of chemotherapy or radiotherapy. The timing of surgery is often crucial and opportunities to perform it can be missed. The aim is not curative but palliative. The cancer will often recur following surgery and occasionally skin closure and healing is a problem because of tumour bulk. Flaps of skin can be taken from the latissimus dorsi and the rectus abdomini muscle in order to improve the chances of skin closure and healing. This is a major surgical procedure (Chapter 9).

The advantages and disadvantages of surgery should be carefully discussed with the woman and she will need time, support information and counselling to be able to make an informed decision. It is the patient's priorities that must be recognized. For some women, the possibility of not having a fungating, perhaps malodorous, wound, that requires regular dressing is an incentive to have surgery, even if their life expectancy is short and they are aware of the potential for the cancer to recur around the incision line.

'Toilet' or salvage mastectomy may be the treatment of choice for women who have presented late with a fungating lesion.

NURSING MANAGEMENT

The lack of research-based literature on the management of malignant fungating lesions poses a problem for nurses and should perhaps encourage everyone to look more closely at this subject. The management of malignant fungating lesions is rarely mentioned or discussed at any length in medical or nursing literature. It is essential for nurses to remember that fungating lesions have a pathological basis: unless this is treated, and the cancer responds to the treatment, healing will not occur. Many forget this and become very frustrated if healing does not occur because the aim has been unrealistic. It is essential that the aims of management are understood by patients, relatives and nurses and that they are realistic in nature. The aim is to promote healing if possible, minimize pain, infection and bleeding, and enhance quality of life within the bounds of what is acceptable to each individual patient.

The assessment

Each lesion requires individual assessment and planning of treatment, which should be realistic and acceptable to the patient and carers. If the treatment does not promote quality of life and a sense of well-being, it should be changed. Few treatments are absolute: when the prognosis is poor, the primary aim should be to promote comfort (Saunders and Regnard, 1989).

Each patient is a unique individual and requires individual assessment and attention to her priorities and needs. The goals should be:

- attainable
- realistic
- acceptable to the patient.

Measure and draw the lesion, noting the main problems it presents and those identified by the patient (Morrison, 1987). Accurate assessment and precise documentation are vital, allowing nurses to monitor the stages of healing and the effectiveness of treatment. However, change in the lesions is usually slow and deterioration often occurs due to progression of the disease. For this reason regular measurements are not usually recommended as lack of progress may lead to disappointment for the patient and nurse.

An understanding of the basic mechanisms of wound-healing is fundamental to the planning of care for each individual wound and is essential for the selection of dressings (Gwyther 1988). The assessment is a dynamic process. Effective management is dependent on an accurate, comprehensive assessment of the patient. Any underlying factors that might influence wound-healing should be noted and appropriate action initiated. Many factors can impair healing and may need investigating, including:

- nutrition
- drug therapies
- disease progression
- other disease, e.g. cardiovascular disease
- infection
- hydration
- allergies
- patient hygiene
- mobility
- patient compliance.

A multidisciplinary approach is essential. The dietician usually has an important role to play as it is often very difficult for these patients to enjoy food with a malodorous wound located often just inches away from their face. Even when the odour is controlled, patients may still sense the underlying smell.

It is important for the nurse to be familiar with the patient's history, previous treatments used and their efficacy, the physical appearance of the lesion, and the patient's description of how it looked before. The nurse needs to document the diameter, depth, colour and odour of the lesion. It is useful to have a photograph of it, although this may prove too distressing for the woman. Actual and potential problems must also be considered, and wound swabs are helpful. The state and extent of the physical symptoms should be noted, including bleeding, infection, odour, exudate and pain.

The nurse must make an informed and considered choice about the use of conventional and non-conventional topical agents and dressings; this is as pertinent to the nursing management of malignant lesions as it is to that of any other wound type (Butler, 1985; Leaper, 1986). Awareness of and sensitivity to the psychological problems that the patient with a malignant lesion may be experiencing is equally as important as the control of physical symptoms (Bennett, 1985). The understanding of the psychological sequence is imperative and is as important as the physical sequence, indeed one cannot be considered without the other: the patient must be treated as a whole.

WOUND MANAGEMENT

The management of fungating lesions is commonly the responsibility of the nurse when medical treatment is no longer appropriate or is ineffective (Ivelic and Lyne, 1990). Nurses need a basic understanding of the wound-healing process and dressings so as to be able to make a considered and appropriate choice of dressing.

The characteristics of the ideal wound dressing are listed below (Draper, 1985; Johnson, 1989). It:

- is non-adherent
- is impermeable to bacteria
- maintains high humidity
- allows removal of excess exudate
- is thermally insulating
- is non-toxic and non-allergenic
- is comfortable
- protects from trauma.

No single dressing satisfies all the criteria, so the wound must be assessed and an informed decision made. Nurses should look at the products available and at research, and should consider the goal in tandem with the patient. It is useful to consider the particular problem areas of fungating lesions to aid in the selection of appropriate topical agents and dressings. The areas to consider are:

- cleansing
- debriding
- odour control
- haemostasis
- dressings
- pain control.

Cleansing

Modern primary dressings greatly reduce the need for wound cleansing because of their hydrophilic effects. Gentle wound cleansing with 0.9% physiological saline is sufficient to remove loose debris and necrotic material (Johnson, 1989). Fungating wounds can often be well managed using a clean technique. It is most beneficial for these patients to cleanse by showering or bathing, particularly as they often feel unclean. When healing is unlikely, treating the wound as 'normally' as possible is most important and may help the patient to view it with less disgust. If bleeding from the lesion is a problem, however, care should be taken when showering as it may induce bleeding.

Research into the treatments used by nurses on fungating lesions (Foltz, 1980; Pugh, 1983; Sims and Fitzgerald, 1985) has revealed the use of a number of agents that have recently received criticism. Evidence suggests that the controlled use of topical antiseptics should be reappraised: it is important for nurses to be aware of the risks associated with cleansing with antiseptics before considering their use. Johnson (1989) identifies these risks as sensitization allergies, bacterial resistance, interference with the normal healing process and damage to the tissues, among others. These principles are relevant to any form of wound management.

The aim of cleansing should be to provide the patient with a sense of freshness, cleanliness and comfort.

Debridement

Debridement is the removal of slough and necrotic tissue from a wound. Bale and Harding (1990) recommend that unless tissue is superficial or hanging loose, nurses should not interfere and remove it. For deep necrotic fungating wounds, surgical debridement is occasionally indicated if the patient's condition is suitable. Only when necrotic and slough areas are removed can the full extent of the wound be recognized. Tissue repair cannot begin until the wound has been fully debrided after which granulation tissue can form and healing by secondary intention will proceed (Bale and Harding, 1987). The removal of necrotic tissue can significantly improve problems relating to excess exudate production and malodour.

Enzymatic agents have the ability to dissolve slough, but the nurse must be skilful when using these. Polysaccharides, hydrogel and hydrocolloids are effective debridants in both necrotic and sloughing wounds without traumatizing the surrounding skin (Johnson, 1989). This is particularly important with fungating lesions as the surrounding skin is usually very fragile. These products have been especially designed to provide a good healing environment: the moist environment allows the necrotic tissue to rehydrate and the separation of damaged tissue to occur.

Odour control

Odour control presents a major challenge to nurses and patients. The odour is caused by the invasion of bacteria; foul smelling odours are associated with anaerobic bacteria. The presence of bacteria in these wounds is inevitable but effective debridement helps reduce the problem. A wound swab should be taken and appropriate antibiotics administered. Metronidazole assists odour control but can cause nausea; this may be reduced by administering it as a suppository. Patients are also advised against taking alcohol as this gives Metronidazole an emetic effect. Abstention from alcohol may conflict with a patient's lifestyle and reduce quality of life and for this reason it may be contraindicated. Topical metronidazole gel is effective in controlling odour. The gel can be applied directly to the wound area, is painless and can have a soothing effect.

Charcoal dressings and air filters fitted with absorbents can be valuable and are worth trying. Some modern dressings now provide a charcoal base. Masking odours with perfumes usually fails as the patient begins to associate the odour with the perfume. The informed use of certain essetial oils has, however, proved useful.

It is important to nurse these patients in a well-ventilated room and to discuss the odour control with them as this area usually causes the greatest anxiety. The patient is living with the smell at close proximity at all times, and even when the odour is controlled the patient is still acutely aware of it. Patients often feel very isolated and are aware that other people can smell the offensive odour. It is important to address this problem and aim to prevent it. Deodorizing oil lamps can be very useful in reducing the odour and many patients find it very helpful in their own homes. Many modern dressings absorb, immobilize and control bacteria.

Haemostasis

Capillary bleeding is a very common problem. Usually it can be controlled by applying gentle pressure. The drying out of dressings should be avoided and if this occurs they should be gently soaked off to prevent capillary bleeding. Alginate dressings have been found to have haemostatic properties but, to date, little research has been carried out using such agents. Silver sulphadiazine has been proved to be effective in controlling capillary bleeding but it has not been scientifically proven as a haemostatic (Fitzgerald and Sims, 1987). Radiotherapy to the area may also be used to control bleeding.

Severe haemorrhage from a fungating breast cancer is uncommon but very alarming (Rankin, Rubens and Redy, 1988). Surgical ligation of the internal mammary artery has been necessary in a few cases. Arterial catheterization and embolization with a number of materials was used successfully by Rankin, Rubens and Redy (1988) to control severe and recurrent haemorrhage from an ulcerating lesion.

Dressings

Comfort, absorption of exudate, odour control and cosmetic appearance need to be considered when choosing a dressing. It is difficult to assess the advantages of many dressings as so many factors contribute to fungating lesions. The use of dry dressings is contraindicated as they adhere to the wounds making removal traumatic, often causing capillary bleeding, and thereby providing a channel for infection to reach the wound (Draper, 1985). The principles of choosing an ideal dressing have been discussed earlier.

Many modern dressings are able to absorb excess exudate, which can cause tremendous problems for the patients. Heavily exudating wounds destroy patients' confidence if the exudate leaks on to clothing. Copious discharge indicates the presence of infection, and these patients can also suffer protein loss and electrolyte imbalance. Nurses and patients must be aware of these potential complications. Excessive exudate also renders the skin even more fragile and protection of healthy tissue is important. Occasionally a barrier cream for the surrounding skin is indicated. Occlusive dressings are often useful in providing control of both exudate and odour. Non-adherent dressings reduce pain, bleeding and destruction of granulating tissue. Bulky dressings can cause both physical and psychological problems and will be discussed later.

Pain control

Pain caused by the application or removal of a wound dressing is seen too frequently in clinical practice. Pain is not inevitable in many instances and is caused by poor technique or the inappropriate selection of wound dressing (Thomas, 1989).

Comfort and pain control are priorities and a careful choice of dressing is essential. Patients may need analgesic support during the changing of dressings; if so it should be administered at an appropriate time beforehand.

Unnecessary pain during the management of a fungating lesion only makes the experience even more distressing for the patient.

NON-CONVENTIONAL WOUND MANAGEMENT

Non-conventional treatments, such as the application of live natural yoghurt, are widely used on fungating lesions. Little information is available about the effectiveness of yoghurt. Welch (1982) suggests that it is the low pH of yoghurt and buttermilk or the lactobacilli that affect the wound or the odour producing micro-organisms in it. Many patients have reported the soothing and deodorizing effect of yoghurt, but research has not yet been carried out to support this practice.

Icing sugar or sugar paste have been reported to have a debriding action (Sims and Fitzgerald, 1985) but information about their mode of action is scarce. Non-conventional therapies are sometimes turned to as a last resort because of the dearth of research-based literature on the nursing management of fungating lesions. However, nurses must be well informed about any side-effects and should discuss the use of non-conventional approaches with medical staff.

PRACTICAL HELP AND ADVICE

Psychological insights support physical care: effective management of both body and mind combine to facilitate the optimum quality of care. Practical aspects are very important: good practice may enhance or improve the patient's quality of life. Individual assessment is essential to establish patient priorities. Practical help is achieved from the basis of knowledge and understanding of the condition and treatments. It is important that information-giving, teaching and counselling are initiated at an early stage.

A flexible attitude to patients' wishes is important. Some women may wish to dress their own wounds rather than waiting for the nurse each day so as to gain greater control over their time and routine. Principles that encourage a good wound care technique should be followed, but they must also be acceptable to the patient. The patient's family may also wish to become involved with day to day care. On the other hand, a patient and her family may not even wish to look at her wound.

The choice of dressing is important. Some women may prefer less bulky dressings, changed frequently, for cosmetic purposes. Other women may consider excessive exudate the bigger problem and feel more confident with bulky dressings. Imagination with clothing choices combined with trial and error is often necessary before a patient's confidence returns.

Often a 'normal' bra is sufficient if it is supportive and comfortable, gives a good shape to the breast and allows dressings to stay in place. However, bras can become uncomfortable, particularly with more extensive lesions. Cotton tubinet vests can be useful for comfort and efficiency. Vest bras are also now availble in many high street stores and offer both support and comfort. They allow the dressing to stay in place without excessive use of tape that damages the often fragile skin. It is important that they are easy to wear as many women have a problem with excessive exudate. In special cases bras need to be made to measure. Confidence will increase if the bra/vest bra allows dressings to remain in place and is comfortable to wear.

The nurses need a good knowledge of prosthetics. A shell prosthesis worn over the fungating lesion facilitates a more equal and natural breast shape. The provision of a prosthesis is occasionally indicated for the opposite side if the fungating lesion protrudes, particularly with bulky dressings.

The nursing approach should be sensitive and realistic in order to enable the woman to wear clothes in which she feels both comfortable and confident. These more positive feelings may lead to some improvement in body image and self-esteem. The woman should be encouraged to feel good about herself again and it is important to aim for this. The woman with a fungating breast lesion may live for many years or for only a short time, always improved quality of life is an objective.

Nurses should also consider the practicalities surrounding the dressing: where the patient will get her supply from? Who will collect and dispose of the used dressings? Is there a suitable laundry service? The smooth running of these practical issues is essential.

THE NURSE'S ROLE

The majority of these patients' care is co-ordinated in the community and the nursing management of fungating lesions is most often the province of the district nurse who must also identify the implications of this condition for the patient's lifestyle and offer support for practical and emotional issues. Good communication between the hospital and the community, and the patient and her family are essential.

For the nurse to care effectively for the patient and her family, she needs to be equipped with a specialist body of knowledge including an understanding of breast cancer, its treatments, factors leading to fungating lesions and their progression. The nurse needs an insight into the physical, psychological, emotional and spiritual consequences, the impact the disease/condition has on the life of the patient and her family and an understanding of altered body image. A knowledge of the actual and potential problems is also required and the nurse should be up to date with wound management techniques and research-based literature pertinent to this area.

The nurse needs to be sensitive, calm and empathetic in her approach. Often a nurse may initially feel critical of the patient for neglecting the signs and symptoms, but it is important not to be judgemental as patients can be very sensitive to the reaction of others. Very good communication skills are essential and information, teaching and counselling should be offered appropriately. Close liaison with the multidisciplinary team should be maintained between the community and hospital nursing staff and the patient and her family to facilitate continuity of care.

PSYCHOSOCIAL CONSIDERATIONS

The diagnosis of breast cancer can have a devastating effect on patients and their families. Between 20% and 40% of women with breast cancer experience some degree of psychological morbidity regardless of treatment modality (Wilkinson, Maguire and Tait, 1988). The diagnosis of metastatic breast cancer can be even more traumatic for a woman and her family than the initial diagnosis (Denton, 1989). Patients in this group have to deal not only with the diagnosis of breast cancer but also with the emotional pain and fear of watching it grow and produce many unacceptable consequences. An awareness of the complexity of the problems patients may be experiencing or have experienced is essential.

Altered body image is a major problem for these patients and is both physical and psychological in nature. Many women experience physical/social and emotional difficulties as a consequence of their fungating lesions and these may lead to the following problems.

1. Altered role within the family – isolation may occur as a result of feelings of fear, guilt, anxiety or disgust. Physical and emotional restrictions may compromise the woman's role within the family unit.
2. Altered role within the community – the woman may feel embarrassed and isolated by a fear of potential problems associated with odour, exudate and bleeding control and the constraints of a bulky dressing. A withdrawal from social functions is not uncommon.
3. Loss of wholeness and attractiveness – the breast can often become unrecognizable and non-functional. The motivation to feel attractive is lost because of the multiple problems with the fungating wound.
4. Loss of control because of the disease – fear of the future and a change in quality of life can lead to anxiety, depression and despair.
5. Sexual dysfunction – this may be physical or psychological in nature. Women may fear rejection if their self-esteem is low, and if they don't consider themselves to be attractive they will not believe others will find them so. These women are often very isolated, many fear even being cuddled or touched because of their own feelings of disgust for the lesion.

The psychological effects may be extreme because of the constant visual reminder. Many women are not close to death and the ability to cope and live with the condition presents a major challenge. Patients must be approached as individuals; care needs to be well-planned and directed in a sensitive manner. Charles-Edwards (1983) illustrates the importance of the nursing approach: 'Much can be done to keep the lesion comfortable and odourless but the attitude with which the dressing is performed will do more to alleviate the patient's feelings of shame, disgust and alienation, than any of these potions!'

The lack of information about malignant lesions leaves nurses to rely on their intuition and experience, however varied that may be (Ivelic and Lyne, 1990), a situation that is often unsatisfactory given the serious nature of this condition. The nurse needs the skills of listening, communication and counselling, and a calm, sensitive, respectful and empathetic approach may help to facilitate the patient's ability to cope. A trusting relationship between the patient, nurse and family must be established.

Privacy is essential for the patients and her relatives and is also important for delicate and skilful interventions by the nurse. Support is dynamic and helping patients to cope with readjusting and adapting to new limitations is imperative. Patients may have many feelings, including guilt, embarrassment, blame, denial, anger, fear, bereavement, anxiety and depression, and they need an environment in which to express these feelings. The implications for other family members are also enormous, and their means of coping is very important; they too need support and guidance and 'permission' to express their feelings. The primary aim for the nurse in counselling these women is to assist them to find their own means of coping with the emotional consequences of their condition.

REFERENCES

Bale, S. and Harding, K. (1987) Fungating breast wounds. *Journal of District Nursing*, **5**(12), 4–5.

Bale, S. and Harding, K. (1990) Using modern dressing to effect debridement. *The Professional Nurse*, 244–8.

Bennett, M. (1985) As normal a life as possible. *Community Outlook*, **81**(7), 35–8.

Blackley, P. (1986) Local Recurrence, in *Complications in the Management of Breast Disease* (ed. R.W. Blaney), Baillière Tindall, Oxford.

Bloom, N.J.G., Richards, W.W. and Harris, E.J. (1962) Natural history of untreated breast cancer. *British Medical Journal*, **2**, 213–21.

Butler, G.A. (1985) Desloughing agents at work. *Nursing Mirror*, **160**(13), 29.

Charles-Edwards, A. (1983) *The Nursing Care of the Dying Patient*, Beaconsfield Limited, Beaconsfield.

Denton, S. (1989) Nursing Patients with Breast Cancer, in *Oncology for Nurses and Health Professionals, Volume 3* (ed. D. Borley), Harper and Row, London.

Doyle, D. (1980) Domiciliary terminal care. *The Practitioner*, **224**(1344), 575–82.

Draper, J. (1985) Making the dressing fit the wound. *Nursing Times*, **81**(41), 32–5.

Fallowfield, L. (1991) *Breast Cancer*, Tavistock/Routledge, London.

Fitzgerald, U. and Sims, R. (1987) A positive approach (wound care). *Community Outlook*, 16–21.

Foltz, A.T. (1980) Nursing care of ulcerating metastatic lesions. *Oncology Nursing Forum*, **7**(2), 8–13.

Gwyther, J. (1988) Skilled dressing. *Nursing Times*, **84**(19), 60–4.

Haagensen, C.D. (1971) *Diseases of the Breast*, 2nd edn, Saunders, Eastbourne.

Ivelic, O. and Lyne, P.A. (1990) Fungating and ulcerating malignant lesions: a review of the literature. *Journal of Advanced Nursing*, **15**, 83–8.

Johnson, A. (1989) Wound management – are you getting it right? *The Professional Nurse*, 306–8.

Kumar, A., Shar, L., Khanna, S. and Khanna, N. (1987) Preoperative chemotherapy for fungating breast cancer. *Journal of Surgical Oncology*, **36**, 295–8.

Leaper, D. (1986) Antiseptics and their effect on healing tissue. *Nursing Times*, **82**(22), 45–7.

Morrison, M. (1987) Priorities in wound management, part 2. *The Professional Nurse*, 402–11.

Petrek, J.A., Glenn, P.D. and Craner, A.R. (1983) Ulcerated breast cancer, patients and outcome. *The American Surgeon*, **49**(4), 187–91.

Pugh, B. (1983) The prodigal son. *Nursing Times*, **79**(23), 70–2.

Rankin, E.M., Rubens, R.D. and Redy, J.F. (1988) Transcatheter embolisation to control severe bleeding in fungating breast cancer. *European Journal of Surgical Oncology*, **14**, 27–32.

Rosen, T. (1980) Cutaneous metastases. *The Medical Clinics of North America*, **64**(5), 885–900.

Saunders, J. and Regnard, C. (1989) Management of malignant ulcers – a flow diagram. *Palliative Medicine*, **3**, 153–5.

Sims, R. and Fitzgerald, V. (1985) *The Community Nursing Management of Patients with Ulcerating/Fungating Disease*, The Royal College of Nursing, London.

Thomas, S. (1989) *Pressure Sores Aetiology. Treatment and Prevention*, Croom Helm, London.

Thomas, S. (1992) Current practices in the management of fungating lesions and radiation damaged skin. *The Surgical Materials Testing Laboratory*, Bridgend, Mid Glamorgan.

Welch, L.B. (1982) Buttermilk and yoghurt odour control of open lesions. *Critical Care Update*, **9**(11), 39–44.

Wilkinson, S., Maguire, G.P. and Tait, A. (1988) Life after breast cancer. *Nursing Times*, **84**(40), 34–7.

Physiotherapy and breast cancer | 13

Clare Sleigh

INTRODUCTION

Physiotherapists can play a large role in the care of patients with breast cancer, helping them with some of the physical problems that may arise, such as the side-effects of medical interventions (e.g. surgery, radiotherapy or chemotherapy) and the effects of the spread of cancer from the breast to other soft tissues or bone.

Physiotherapy assists patients in a physical way, via exercises or walking aids such as sticks or crutches, for example, but also encompasses the giving of advice and educating patients about relevant aspects of their condition, such as how and when to start lifting after breast surgery. It is therefore important for physiotherapists to have full access to patients' medical records and a good knowledge of the pathology and management of breast cancer so as to be able to answer patients' queries confidently.

Physiotherapy is always more effective if the treatment is begun early. Easy access to the physiotherapist is therefore essential but can only be achieved if there are good lines of communication within the multidisciplinary team, including among doctors, nurses, occupational therapists and social workers. Physiotherapists must also be ready to refer patients to other professionals for their help and advice. In these ways the patient and her relatives may receive the best possible care and support at all stages.

BREAST SURGERY

Most patients undergoing breast surgery require physiotherapy afterwards to help them maximize their functional ability. At the Royal Marsden Hospital, usually physiotherapists consider it necessary as a routine to see patients undergoing certain breast surgery, which requires the nursing and medical staff to refer such patients to them pre-operatively.

Patients undergoing axillary dissection, mastectomy or surgery involving implant or tissue transplantation need shoulder exercises to enable them to recover a full range of movement in the arm post-operatively. Wingate (1985) has shown that patients who do not receive post-mastectomy arm exercises lose a significant amount of movement in the shoulder. Patients tend to keep their arm by their side unless they are actively encouraged to move it and overcome the unnatural sensations this elicits after surgery. Interestingly, Wingate also noted that patients who had undergone an operation on the side of their dominant hand/arm achieved a greater range of movement in the early post-operative phase; he suggested that this may be due to the greater functional reliance being put on this arm.

Close liaison with the surgical team and nursing staff is always important so that special instructions can be followed and any problems can be reported and acted on quickly. Problems are minimized, however, when post-operative exercises are undertaken in a controlled fashion and monitored carefully by a physiotherapist.

Pre-operative physiotherapy

Whenever possible, the physiotherapist should assess the patient pre-operatively. This assessment should include the following:

- Details of the patient's previous medical history, history of the present condition to include any previous surgery, radiotherapy and chemotherapy.
- Details of the patient's home situation, family support, type of occupation, leisure activities and hand dominance. This allows a greater understanding of the patient's fears about the impact of the operation on her everyday life, and the treatment regime can be modified to allow for the patient's individual needs. This knowledge will lead to better teamwork between therapist and patient, which ensures more patient satisfaction and a better functional outcome.
- A physical evaluation of the shoulder joint. After the majority of operations we would expect the patient to regain her full range of movement in the shoulder complex. However, if range of movement was severely limited pre-operatively it should be explained to the patient that although this range will be regained, a normal range of movement may never again be achieved. There are exceptions to this, of course. A woman who has lost a few degrees of movement only recently, for example after a course of radiotherapy, would be expected to regain a full range of movement, but she should be advised that it may take longer and she should continue her exercises with perhaps greater diligence than some other patients.

- Observation of the posture of the shoulder and whole body. Although the breast is a small area of the woman's body, surgery can affect her whole posture post-operatively. This can lead to a variety of seemingly unrelated problems later in the recovery, such as neck pain, even years after the operation, if it is not corrected quickly.

Post-operative physiotherapy

Each patient is reassessed by a physiotherapist on her first post-operative day. Firstly, the patient is questioned about her general state, level of pain and level of activity. It is not unusual to find that she has already brushed her hair using the affected arm, which is a great morale booster, and other activities may also have been undertaken, such as eating breakfast. Pain is occasionally a problem, in which case the physiotherapist should arrange to treat the patient approximately half an hour after analgesia has been administered to minimize any discomfort experienced.

Secondly, the operation site is observed as closely as possible by the physiotherapist. If the patient has had axillary dissection she will often have had her dressings taken down and replaced by a clear dressing after the breast drain has been removed, in which case it is easy to observe the extent of the incision, the amount of exudate under the dressing and whether there is any evidence of infection in the area.

Next the exercises should be explained to the patient. Modifications in the regime for the different types of surgery are explained later in this chapter. The patient is given a sheet of exercises (Figure 13.1) with specific instructions for her to follow. If problems are encountered, such as wound infections, modifications can be made, but for the majority of women it is sufficient for them to perform the exercises on the sheet to regain full range of shoulder movement and optimum arm function. The patient reads the instructions while the physiotherapist demonstrates the exercise, indicating the salient points. The physiotherapist then watches while the patient performs the exercise, correcting position and giving an indication of the level of performance that is desired so as to avoid letting the patient move her arm too far or not far enough.

The main factor limiting shoulder movement in this early phase of recovery is a sensation of tension in the incision and surrounding musculature. Because this is a subjective sensation each patient will find her own individual limit to movement. Comparisons between patients should not be encouarged, but the physiotherapist should expect her to achieve at least 45° of shoulder elevation on the first post-operative day. If the patient cannot move her arm this far she should be verbally encouraged to gain further range, but she should never be physically pushed past her self-set limit because of the greatly increased risk of trauma.

There is usually a reason for a seemingly poor patient performance. It may be related to the operative procedure or the position of the wound drains,

Department of Physiotherapy Arm Exercises

SET A - to be performed in sitting ... times a day.

1. Hand on shoulder - lift elbow out to side and down.
2. Hand on shoulder - lift elbow forwards and down.
3. Clasp hands behind neck, keeping head straight - stretch elbows to the side and back to the middle.
4. Put hand behind back - reach up back as far as possible.

Do each exercise ... times each session.

SET B - to be performed in sitting ... times a day.

1. Lift straight arm forwards above head.
2. Lift straight arm sideways and continue up towards head.

Do each exercise ... times each session. Continue these exercises for ...

SET C - to be performed lying down ... times a day.

Hold each position for a count of 10.

1. Arm by side - lift arm forwards above head keeping elbow straight. Give a gentle push with other arm to gain extra movement.
2. Arm by side - lift arm out sideways and continue up towards head.
3. Clasp hands behind neck - slowly lower elbows out to the side to touch the bed.

These exercises are useful if your shoulder becomes stiff for any reason.

Do each exercise ... times each session.

Figure 13.1 Arm exercises.

in which case it will settle with time or when the drain is removed, or the patient may be experiencing more pain because of her heightened perception to any sensation in this situation. In this case other methods must be used to reassure the patient and gain her confidence; these could include returning later in the day to supervise the exercises, or re-explaining the exercise technique.

EXERCISE REGIMES

The arm exercises have been designed to enable patients to regain their pre-operative range of shoulder movement as soon as possible without causing wound complications. Their functions are explained below.

Set A

These exercises are performed by patients with a wound drain *in situ*. They are a short lever type, which means they are done with a flexed elbow, thus reducing the forces acting across the shoulder joint and so reducing the

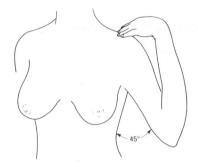

Figure 13.2 Set A exercises are for the patient with a drain *in situ*.

stress on the incision (Scott, 1975). The majority of women will gain
45° of abduction in the initial session with minimal increase in discomfort (Figure 13.2). The exercises are designed to move the glenohumeral
joint and shoulder girdle through four planes and prepare the shoulder
complex for a full range of movement when the wound drains are removed
(Gray, 1980). Minimal stress is put on the incision because the exercises are done actively, allowing reciprocal relaxation of the muscles
on the inferior aspect of the joint, and the patient is in full control throughout.

Exercise 1 works the abductor muscles and stretches soft tissue on the
inferior aspect of the joint and in the axilla.

Exercise 2 works the shoulder flexors and scapula rotators, while stretching
the shoulder extensors.

Exercise 3 uses both arms to stretch the soft tissue across the anterior
aspect of the chest and encourages lateral rotation. This is a very important
movement because if lateral rotation of the humerus is restricted, full elevation
will be limited since the greater tuberosity will not be able to clear the acromion
process.

Exercise 4 works the medial rotators and is the classic manoeuvre used
by women to do up their bras.

Set A is performed four times a day, usually around meal times so that
the patient has something to jog her memory. Each exercise is repeated four
times at each session.

Set B

These exercises are started when the drains are removed. They are performed
in a sitting position and with an extended elbow. This progression allows the

patient to move her shoulder through a greater range and increase the weight lifted by the muscles as a result of the longer lever moving around the fulcrum of the glenohumeral joint (Hollis, 1976). A typical home exercise programme would be a warm-up using set A and then four repetitions of set B, done twice a day.

The patient returns to clinic after approximately two weeks. She should see a physiotherapist who will check her range of movement and question her about her level of activity and any problems she may be experiencing with the exercises. Some of the problems that may occur in this period, such as seroma or wound infection will necessitate the alteration of the exercise programme.

If the patient is progressing uneventfully she should now have reached three-quarters of the full range of movement at her shoulder, and be following her regime of exercises twice daily. Once the sutures are removed she will usually gain full range of movement, and will need no further supervision from the physiotherapist. She is advised to continue her exercises twice a day for a further month and thereafter to check the range of shoulder movement in a mirror daily for a further two months. This will enable her to notice quickly any deterioration in range when she could contact the physiotherapy department for further advice or instructions.

Set C

Set C exercises are not taught routinely to post-operative patients because their function is to stretch the soft tissues around the joint and they could cause damage if done too early on after the operation. These exercises are only used once the sutures have been removed if the wound is healing and the patient has developed a stiff shoulder.

Exercise 1 stretches the tissues on the inferior aspect of the glenohumeral joint. Gravity works to assist the flexor muscles with the patient in a lying position. The patient can assist her arm into further elevation by pushing with her other hand on the affected elbow. The stretch applied must be slow and sustained rather than short and bouncing in nature, to avoid damage to the muscles or ligaments. Each position is held for 10 seconds and repeated five times.

Exercise 2 is performed lying on her side, but the principles are the same. The shoulder is moved through abduction to alter the stretch on the ligaments from exercise 1.

Exercise 3 stretches the anterior of the joint and allows the patient to gain more lateral rotation. It is performed while lying supine and additional pressure can be given by the patient pushing her elbow further into range with her other hand.

MODIFICATIONS FOR RECONSTRUCTIVE SURGERY

When the patient has a subpectoral implant the surgeon may restrict the range of movement at the shoulder to 90° (shoulder level) for the first three months after the operation. The physiotherapist will teach the patient the exercises in sets A and B, but will limit the range to shoulder level. Three months after the operation the patient will be recalled for a physiotherapy assessment to review her shoulder movement. If any problem is observed, or the patient has any complaints about her arm function, she can be taught exercises to continue at home or she can attend for a short course of physiotherapy as necessary.

The patients who have had a muscle flap will progress slowly because of the dangers of moving the flap on its vascular bed and disrupting the blood supply. The physiotherapist will delay starting exercises until she has established that the flaps are healthy and viable, and that any movement will not have any adverse effects.

IMMEDIATE POST-OPERATIVE COMPLICATIONS

The post-operative recovery is not always straightforward and it is worthwhile considering when physiotherapy may need to be modified.

Seroma

Collections of fluid around the operation site are not uncommon. They may be removed by aspiration and the area then observed. Research has tried to discover the influence the timing of post-operative exercises has on the amount of wound drainage and seroma formation after mastectomy and axillary dissection. Flew (1979) found that wound drainage could be decreased if the arm was totally immobilized post-operatively for seven days before starting physiotherapy. Rodier et al. (1987), however, compared early with delayed physiotherapy and found no significant difference in wound drainage or the incidence of seroma formation. Hence, in many centres, physiotherapists commence mobilization of the shoulder from the first post-operative day. If the patient does present with a seroma the physiotherapist's role is to monitor how active the patient is being with her arm and to give advice on a sensible level of activity for her stage in the recovery period. It is not unusual for patients to be so pleased with their progress in the hospital that when they get home, and are faced with a family to look after, they do not realize how much more they are using their arm. A gentle reminder to increase activities slowly and carefully is helpful.

Wound infection

Occasionally the patient will develop increased pain, heat and redness around the incision, which usually indicates that they have a wound infection. Exercises are stopped and the arm is rested to minimize movement and the spread of the infection via the bloodstream and compromised lymphatic system. Infections encourage the later development of lymphoedema and it is important that they are treated quickly.

Wound breakdown

Wound breakdown after reconstructive surgery occurs most commonly because of a compromised blood supply to the muscle flap. When this happens exercises are stopped and the physiotherapist should liaise with the surgical team about the course of action that is proposed. This could include an immediate surgical salvage procedure, in which case the physiotherapist will reassess the patient post-operatively and continue the rehabilitation from this point. Occasionally the surgical team will decide to wait and observe the wound to discover the full extent of the necrosis; physiotherapy exercises will usually cease during this period.

Long thoracic nerve palsy

Very occasionally the long thoracic nerve which supplies the serratus anterior muscle can be damaged during surgery. The patient will report difficulty in pushing manoeuvres and when the physiotherapist observes the scapula he or she will notice the classic winging deformity. Treatment for this problem involves teaching the patient to stretch the shoulder passively daily to prevent contractures and advising on movements to overcome the functional limitations. Referral to an occupational therapist can be beneficial. The patient is also advised to monitor the problem so that if the nerve begins to recover she can return for a course of physiotherapy.

LATE POST-OPERATIVE COMPLICATIONS REQUIRING PHYSIOTHERAPY

'Cording'

This is a phenomenon that occurs after axillary dissection which causes limitation of movement and pain. Unfortunately, little is known about its cause. Clinically the patient will report a sudden increase in pain in her axilla, spreading into the breast proximally and down the medial aspect of the arm distally. This pain is worse when the arm is raised because of the tethering effect of the 'cords'. On palpation, bands of fibrous tissue can be felt, especially when they are stretched by putting the arm into a position of shoulder elevation, elbow and wrist extension. The limitation of movement experienced will indicate the severity of the condition and in the worst cases patients are unable to raise their arm above shoulder level without first flexing their elbow.

Physiotherapy intervention involves stretching exercises, which should be started as quickly as possible after the onset of the 'cording', with analgesic cover if the patient requires it. Pain will diminish as the 'cords' stretch and the range of movement increases, and the patient usually regains full movement in her arm eventually. If the patient has not presented in the physiotherapy department until a while after the 'cords' have developed, recovery will be slower, and she may always have a slight limitation of movement because the fibrous bands become stronger and less extensible as they become more chronic.

Shoulder pain

Patients are often referred with shoulder pain and limitation of movement that are causing problems with the activities of daily living. The causes of these pains are legion, but in every case the basis for an effective course of physiotherapy is an initial assessment where a detailed verbal history is taken, as well as observation of the cervical and thoracic spine, shoulder girdle and glenohumeral joint.

One common cause of shoulder pain is that some patients only continue to exercise until they have a good functional range of movement – enabling them to hang out their washing, for example – but they give up and tolerate the loss of the last few degrees of movement, which they only find to be an inconvenience when, for example, they try to reach an item on a high shelf. In the long run this situation causes muscle and ligament imbalance around the shoulder joint, which can cause a range of different pains. Physiotherapy treatments are particularly useful because they work to stretch the soft tissues around the joint at the limit of range using accessory movements (Maitland, 1983).

Another cause of shoulder pain is an alteration in the patient's posture. After the operation she may be more aware of her breast and will subconsciously protract her shoulder to protect the area. Even though this new position may be only a slight alteration on the normal, held over a prolonged period of time it will cause pain because of the imbalance in joint mechanics, especially on the acromioclavicular joint (Boissonnault and Janos, 1989). Maitland mobilization techniques are an excellent method of treatment for this problem.

RADIOTHERAPY

Radiotherapy is commonly used in conjunction with surgery to improve the survival rates of patients with breast cancer. Rytov and Blichert-Toft (1983) have shown that radiotherapy has a detrimental effect on shoulder mobility in patient's undergoing mastectomy, Swedborg and Wallgreen (1981) demonstrated that a significant decrease in range of movement occurred whether the patient received the radiotherapy pre- or post-mastectomy compared with patients who had a mastectomy only. Both trials demonstrate the need for exercises to prevent loss of function if the patient has received radiotherapy, because soft tissues within the radiation field are prone to fibrosis that can manifest itself nine months to two years after the completion of the treatment. The patient notices a gradual decrease in the amount of movement in her shoulder as the tissues in her axilla fibrose and contract, probably discovering this as an inability to reach objects on a shelf that had previously been accessible. It is a painless process at first, but as the imbalance around the shoulder increases aches and pains develop.

Prophylactic advice is an important part of physiotherapy treatment. When a patient commences radiotherapy a physiotherapist should discuss the importance of her continuing the exercise regime for up to two years after the course of treatment has finished. Patient compliance is increased if the reason the exercises are necessary is discussed, so a brief explanation of the side effects of radiotherapy and the effect of stretching exercises to maintain tissue extensibility should be given. The physiotherapist may also discuss a course of action for the patient to follow if she does notice problems in the future. The plan usually consists of intensifying her stretching exercises and contacting a doctor to gain an early referral to a physiotherapy department, rather than waiting until the fibrous tissue becomes older and more difficult to treat adequately.

A side effect of radiotherapy is desquamation of epithelial cells. When the skin reaction is mild there is little to effect the physiotherapy, but in more severe cases the patient may find the movement of her arm against her body extremely painful. She may then be advised to stop her exercises temporarily and to restart them when the skin reaction settles down. Post-radiation fibrosis can affect the capillaries in the area, causing a disruption in the blood supply to the axilla, breast and arm. Electrical modalities, such as heat or ultrasound, therefore have no place in the treatment of post-radiotherapy fibrosis since they rely on a normal blood supply to dissipate any heat that may be generated; the disruption to the capillaries caused by the radiation means that the effects of the treatments are uncertain.

Brachial plexus lesions

The nerves of the brachial plexus pass through the axilla and can be susceptible to radiation damage, causing alterations in sensation and muscle power in the arm. The specific area of the arm that is affected will depend on the extent of the irradiation to the brachial plexus. The situation may be complicated by the fibrosis of soft tissues, causing limitation in the range of movement at the shoulder. Today, awareness of this as a potential problem following radiotherapy, sometimes occuring months or years after treatment, has led to techniques and practices changing in the delivery of radiotherapy to this area.

Physiotherapy for patients with brachial plexus problems aims to:

- Maintain the range of movements
  The patient is taught exercises to be done daily that take all the affected joints through a full range of movement to maintain the extensibility of the ligaments and muscles. If she cannot do this actively, the patient or a relative is taught to move the joint passively to prevent contractures from forming. Splints may be necessary to prevent contractures and support the joint in a good position; for example, a hand splint may be made for use at night to prevent accidental damage to unprotected finger joints.
- Maintain and increase muscle power

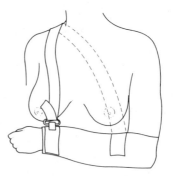

Figure 13.3 A sling to ease pain in shoulder ligaments by supporting the weight of the arm.

Where possible strengthening exercises are performed actively against a resistance, such as a weight or gravity.

- Control pain

This can take many forms depending on what is causing the patient to experience the pain. If the muscles around the shoulder are weak, the weight of the arm tends to pull on the shoulder ligaments causing pain. This situation can be corrected by periodically supporting the weight of the arm in a sling (Figure 13.3). Another cause of pain is the increasing fibrosis in the nerves that causes them to fire abnormal impulses to the brain where the stimuli are interpreted as pain. Transcutaneous electrical nerve stimulation (TENS) can be very helpful in this situation (Frampton, 1988). It is a non-invasive method of analgesia that the patient can control. It is important that the physiotherapist initially gives the patient a great deal of help and advice in the use of the TENS unit to allow her to explore its full potential.

CHEMOTHERAPY

Patients are undergoing increasingly complex chemotherapy regimes for both primary breast disease and metastatic spread and there are many ways in which a physiotherapist may use his or her expertise to minimize the effects of a variety of common side-effects. Most courses of chemotherapy are undertaken on an out-patient basis, so patients who are admitted for treatment are likely to be the more debilitated, with an advanced or aggressive disease, undergoing a more intensive regime. The patient may spend long periods in bed during the worst phase of the chemotherapy when she may be afflicted with symptoms such as nausea, vomiting, diarrhoea and fatigue. This will lead to a decrease in her exercise tolerance as well as predipose her to the other problems of immobility, such as thrombosis and chest infection.

Physiotherapists can minimize the ill-effects of this period of bed-rest by instigating a regime of maintenance exercises for the patient and monitoring her performance. Once the patient begins to mobilize again the physiotherapist can help by assessing her for any areas of weakness, teaching strengthening exercises, monitoring the progress of her mobility, assisting with the provision of relevant walking aids, and giving encouragement as the patient regains her fitness. The aim is to encourage the patient to regain her optimal level of activity.

The second problem that may be encountered is one of respiratory complications. A chest infection can develop when a patient is immunosuppressed, either because she becomes predisposed to a range of opportunistic infections, or as a result of her developing areas of pulmonary atelectasis, which predispose her to the development of a chest infection.

The initial aim of physiotherapy will be to prevent the patient from developing pulmonary atelectasis by encouraging her to change position frequently. Position changes should include alternate side-lying, which, by allowing the abdominal contents to fall away from the diaphram, will reverse the process of alveolar collapse (Hough, 1984; Crosbie and Myles, 1985). These position changes must be accompanied by deep breathing exercises which aid lung re-expansion. If the patient does develop a chest infection, more intensive physiotherapy techniques may be required, including postural drainage, breathing exercises, percussion and coughing, but will always depend on the individual situation.

Rarely a patient may develop a neuropathy because of the effect of the chemotherapeutic agent on the nerves. The problem usually affects the distal part of the nerve, progressing proximally to hands and feet. If a motor nerve is involved muscle weakness can be observed, such as a drop-foot deformity. Physiotherapy can help by maintaining muscle power with active exercises and maintaining function with the provision of walking aids or splints, such as a drop-foot splint. If a sensory nerve is involved the patient may complain of poor sensation over an area of skin and have less appreciation of heat, cold and pressure. She should be advised to take extra precautions to prevent damage, which could include using her elbow to test water temperatures rather than her fingers.

Another rare later side-effect of some chemotherapeutic agents, for example 5-fluorouracil, is the development of a myopathy. The problem presents as increasing muscle weakness and lack of co-ordination and the patient may complain of dropping objects or stumbling more frequently. The aim of physiotherapy is similar to that for patients with neuropathies. There is no problem with altered sensation, but a greater emphasis on exercise and the use of aids helps the patient to overcome her increasing muscle weakness.

BONE METASTASES

Breast cancer frequently metastasizes to bone. The patient may experience pain and be more susceptible to fracture because of the osteolytic nature of the metastases. Spread of the cancer cells is via the bloodstream; the rich blood supply to bone marrow means the bones most affected by metastatic spread are the long bones and the vertebral column. Medical treatments include radiotherapy, chemotherapy and surgical fixation.

Physiotherapy can be useful in the early stages of the metastatic spread when the patient is complaining of pain that may affect her lifestyle. The patient benefits from advice on mobility and postures that will minimize the mechanical stresses across the affected bone. Walking aids, such as crutches and sticks, may be given to decrease the load on the metastasis if the femur or spinal column are involved, and a soft collar or temporary corset may help to minimize the pain in the cervical or lumbar spine. Exercises that will increase the strength and efficiency of the muscles working over the affected bone and joints can be taught. The patient should be encouraged to remain as independent as possible and should be referred to the occupational therapy department for assessment.

Pathological fractures

The physiotherapy for patients who present with a fracture depends on whether the medical treatment selected is surgical or conservative.

Operative repair

Surgical fixation of the fracture site usually allows for rapid post-operative mobilization but the timescale for each patient depends on the surgeon's preference as well as other individual factors, such as the patient's general condition. Good communication within the multidisciplinary team facilitates efficient progress in the patient's rehabilitation.

Physiotherapy helps to increase the patient's mobility with exercises to strengthen muscles and increase the range of movement, advice on activities of daily living and the provision of slings, corsets or walking aids where necessary. Continual assessment of progress will be necessary. The walking aids used by patients with a lower limb fracture will change to reflect their progress. Each patient has a different lifestyle and her level of activity will also be different; a physiotherapist must be able to respond to differing needs. a woman may be keen to go up and down the stairs even though she is non-weight bearing on crutches. Another woman, however, may prefer to have her bed moved downstairs in her house to avoid having to climb the stairs until she is more advanced in her rehabilitation.

Conservative management

Occasionally the patient is managed medically using radiotherapy or chemotherapy for pain control. In these cases physiotherapy aims to optimize the patient's mobility and independence. The provision of a walking aid, such as crutches or a frame, to patients with a lower limb fracture will allow them to mobilize soon after the incident without increasing the pain in their leg. It is important that patients spend as little time as possible in bed, where they quickly develop muscle atrophy and their exercise tolerance drops, making mobilization increasingly difficult.

Patients with a fracture of the vertebral column need specialized care. Stability must be ensured before mobilization is undertaken, because of the high risk of damaging the spinal cord and causing a paraplegia (Dunn, 1983). This is achieved conservatively with the provision of a hard collar, neck brace or permanent corset. These are made to fit the individual because they are intended to support the spinal column as well as immobilize it. When a support is worn continuously the muscles will atrophy through disuse, their action is supersceded by the corset or collar and it is vitally important that the patient is taught to do isometric exercises, such as static abdominal exercises, to maintain or improve the muscle tone or strength.

Physiotherapy can be an important adjunct to the medical forms of pain control in a variety of ways. These include the use of TENS and, in the case of a fracture of the humerus, the provision of a sling to support the weight of the arm and minimize movement at the fracture site, thereby decreasing the pain experienced by the patient. Patients often report that another benefit of a sling is that they feel that their injury is more obvious and so people are less likely to touch their arm or jostle them in a crowd, which helps to prevent sudden and severely painful movements. However, one problem with a sling is that it tends to discourage patients from moving their arm, which predisposes them to joint stiffness, contractures, loss of movement and loss of function. Whenever a sling is administered it should be accompanied by exercises and a lengthy set of instructions and advice from the physiotherapist aimed at maintaining the joint ranges and muscle power while minimizing the pain experienced during the manoeuvres.

Spinal cord compression

The onset of neurological impairment because of pressure on the spinal cord is a not uncommon sequela of vertebral bone metastases. It may manifest as pain, altered sensation and decreasing muscle power below the level of the spinal cord compression. In the most severe cases the patient may develop a paraplegia. A course of radiotherapy to the affected area of the spine is frequently given as treatment together with the medication dexamethazone, a steroid preparation.

Physiotherapy is important for patients with neurological deficit, and the initial assessment allows the physiotherapist to analyse the very specific problems that must be overcome to allow for maximum patient independence. Joints that are immobile because the muscles are denervated must be moved through a full range passively every day. These passive movements are done to prevent contractures which, if allowed to develop, will interfere with the patient's daily living; for example, if a contracture of the tendo calcaneus (Achillis) is allowed to develop the patient will have difficulty keeping her feet on the wheelchair footplate and she will be at a greatly increased risk of damage if her foot slips off. Where the muscles are still innervated, active exercises should be taught to increase the muscle strength. The arms and muscles of the trunk must be strong to allow the patient to use the aids and appliances which will help to maintain her mobility and maximize her independence. The involvement of the occupational therapist at this stage will help to ensure that suitable aids to daily living are supplied to the patient.

The provision of a wheelchair has many implications for the patient: can she transfer herself in and out of it? Will it fit through the doors in her home? It is important that all members of the multidisciplinary team are fully involved in the decision to provide a wheelchair to ensure that it is of benefit to the patient.

Improvements in the patient's condition can occur over a long period of time (Chatterton, 1988) and so rehabilitation can be of great benefit and support to the patient over a similarly long timescale. It is also worth remembering that these patients may be elderly and may therefore need more time, not only for their physical rehabilitation but also for the mental adjustment to their altered situation.

CEREBRAL METASTASES

Breast cancer can metastasize to the brain. The signs and symptoms will depend on the actual site of the metastatic spread and will vary widely from physical manifestations such as ataxia, to perceptual problems such as steroagnosis. Medical treatments include chemotherapy, radiotherapy and steroids. They aim to decrease any cerebral oedema and arrest the growth of the tumour in the confined space of the skull, thereby decreasing pressure on structures of the brain and minimizing the symptoms. It is not unusual for the patient to have a rapid initial decrease in the severity of her symptoms, sometimes in just a matter of hours, especially with the use of anti-inflammatory drugs.

Physiotherapy for these patients is as diverse as the manifestations of the metastases. Some patients may be confused, causing them to have difficulty in interpreting instructions. The physiotherapist must be aware of this problem and other people, such as relatives, can be included in the rehabilitation to help reinforce the treatment.

The patient may also present with physical problems such as poor balance and coordination. Once the extent and nature of the neurological deficit has been assessed by the physiotherapist, exercises to retrain balance or re-educate gait, for example, can be given. Walking aids may be necessary to assist the patient to mobilize as independently and safely as possible.

CONCLUSION

This review of physiotherapy demonstrates the varied input and support that this profession can give to the patient with breast cancer. The emphasis of physiotherapy treatment is to optimize the patient's independence, allowing her to become in some way less reliant on other people and hence improve her quality of life. This aim is achieved not only with the provision of equipment, such as a frame or TENS unit, but also by ensuring that the patient is allowed access to information about her condition. Education of the patient and her family will allow them to become fully involved members of the rehabilitation team and give the patient the confidence to help control her own care, thereby discouraging an over-reliance on supervision by the physiotherapist.

REFERENCES

Boissonnault, W.G. and Janos, S.C. (1989) Dysfunction, Evaluation and Treatment of the shoulder, in *Orthopaedic Physical Therapy* (eds R. Donatelli and M.J. Wooden), Churchill Livingstone, Edinburgh.

Chatterton, P. (1988) Physiotherapy for the terminally ill. *Physiotherapy*, **74**(1), 42–6.

Crosbie, W.J. and Myles, S. (1985) An investigation into the effect of postural modification on some aspects of normal pulmonary function. *Physiotherapy*, **71**(7), 311–14.

Dunn, H.K. (1983) Tumours in the Thoracic and Lumbar Spine, in *Surgery of the Musculoskeletal System Volume 2* (eds I. Evarts and C. McCollister), Churchill Livingstone, Edinburgh.

Flew, T.J. (1979) Wound drainage following radical mastectomy: the effect of restriction of shoulder movement. *British Journal of Surgery*, **66**, 302–5.

Frampton, V. (1988) Transcutaneous Electrical Nerve Stimulation and Chronic Pain, in *Pain: Management and Control in Physiotherapy* (eds P.E. Wells, V. Frampton and D. Bowsher), Heinemann Physiotherapy, London.

Gray, H. (1980) *Gray's Anatomy* 36th edn (eds P.L. Williams and R. Warwick), pp. 456–60, Longman, London.

Hollis, M. (1976) Simple Machines, in *Practical Exercise Therapy* (ed. M. Hollis), Blackwell Scientific Publications, Oxford.

Hough, A. (1984) The effect of posture on lung function. *Physiotherapy*, **70**(3), 101–4.

Maitland, G.D. (1983) Treatment of the glenohumeral joint by passive movement. *Physiotherapy*, **69**(1), 3–7.

Rodier, J.F., Gadonneix, P., Dauplat, J. *et al.* (1987) Influence of the timing of physiotherapy upon the lymphatic complications of axillary dissection for breast cancer. *International Surgery*, **72**, 166–9.

Ryttov, N. and Blichert-Toft, M. (1983) Influence of adjuvant irradiation on shoulder joint function after mastectomy for breast carcinoma. *Acta Radiologica Oncology*, **22**(1), 29.

Scott, P.M. (1975) Mechanics, in *Clayton's Electrotherapy and Actinotherapy*, 7th edn (ed. P.M. Scott), Baillière Tindall, London.

Swedborg, I. and Wallgreen, A. (1981) The effect of pre- and postmastectomy radiotherapy on the degree of edema, shoulder-joint mobility, and gripping force. *Cancer*, **47**, 877–81.

Wingate, L. (1985) Efficacy of physical therapy for patients who have undergone mastectomies. *Physical Therapy*, **65**(6), 896–900.

The management of lymphoedema

14

Caroline Badger

INTRODUCTION

Lymphoedema is defined as 'tissue swelling due to a failure of lymph drainage' (Mortimer, 1990). The lymphatic system is made up of lymph vessels, lymph nodes and lymph itself. The lymph vessels begin in the superficial network as blind-ended capillaries. Water, food and oxygen leave the blood at capillary level to nourish and bathe the tissues. Much of the water, normally about 90%, is reabsorbed at the venous end of the capillaries. The remaining 10% of the water, together with waste materials and large proteins not reabsorbed by the blood, moves from the tissues into the lymph capillaries and is transported along the peripheral pre-collector vessels into the larger lymph collectors.

While the movement of lymph through the peripheral lymphatics is largely dependent on the stimulus provided by local tissue movement, the walls of the lymph collectors are able to contract and thus pump lymph through the system after which it finally drains back into the venous system via the thoracic ducts. Valves in the lymph vessels ensure that lymph flows in one direction only. On its way through the lymphatic network lymph is filtered by a series of lymph nodes.

Lymph drainage commonly fails in breast cancer patients as a result of damage to lymph nodes by surgery and/or radiotherapy, or because of the obstructive effects of local tumour. A study carried out in 1986 (Kissen *et al.*, 1986), recorded an incidence of lymphoedema of 25% in 200 patients following treatment of breast cancer. The incidence rose to 38% in patients who had received both surgery and radiotherapy to the axilla.

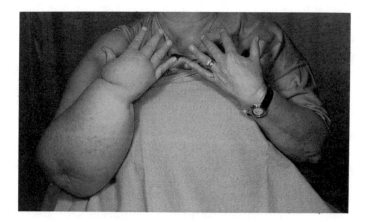

Figure 14.1 Breast cancer-related lymphoedema of the upper limb.

Once obstruction has occurred, an increased burden is placed on the remaining functioning lymphatics. Although the amount of fluid in the tissues (the load on the lymphatics) is not increased, the number of drainage routes is diminished and the resulting backlog of fluid manifests itself as swelling. Swelling does not necessarily appear immediately after cancer treatment; it has been known to appear 20 or even 30 years after the original treatment, even when there is no sign of recurrent disease. In breast cancer patients, swelling may affect any part of the treated upper quadrant of the body but most commonly affects the arm (Figure 14.1).

It is not clear why some people develop lymphoedema after the treatment of breast cancer and others do not. Lymphatics have the ability to regenerate, but this regeneration is inhibited by the extensive scarring that results from surgery and radiotherapy. This threatens the establishment of satisfactory collateral lymph drainage.

When it first appears, swelling may be intermittent and affect only part of the arm, such as the upper arm or hand. The oedema is usually soft and pitting to begin with and often goes down overnight. Some patients can point to a specific event that appeared to precipitate swelling, such as an insect bite on the arm, a cellulitis, or engaging in sudden exertion such as mowing the lawn or carrying something heavy.

As the oedema persists and becomes established, the high protein concentration of the stagnant lymph results in fibrosis of the subcutaneous tissues of the affected area. The thickened tissues cause natural skin folds to become deepened, around the wrist, for example, and the oedema becomes more difficult to pit and less likely to go down overnight. The arm may become distorted in shape and the increase in the size and weight of the limb often results in joint and muscle strain. Local immunity is compromised and recurrent acute inflammmatory episodes are common.

The psychological difficulties of coming to terms with the distortion in size and shape of the arm are by no means negligible. The patient may be reluctant to socialize and may have given up activities that expose the arm, such as swimming. Summer is a particularly difficult time of year for patients with lymphoedema: while they may be able to disguise their breast surgery, it is not so easy to disguise a swollen arm in summer clothes, particularly since the warmer temperatures usually mean an increase in the swelling. Lymphoedema is a constant and visible reminder of the cancer which is difficult for the patient to ignore. Many women find it tiresome and distressing to deal with the almost inevitable 'What have you done to your arm?' question when meeting people for the first time.

While there is at present no cure for lymphoedema, it is possible to reduce the size of the arm and, in patients free of active cancer, to control the swelling long-term. Management of the condition relies on conservative, physical therapies (surgery is rarely indicated and the results are disappointing more often than not), and success is dependent to a large extent on the patient's motivation and compliance. On the whole, patients with lymphoedema form an extremely well-motivated group, particularly when they start to see improvement, but they need a great deal of encouragement and support to comply with treatment on a long-term basis.

Lymphoedema should be treated at the first sign of swelling. At this stage it is relatively easy to treat and patients respond extremely well, occasionally being able to do without a compression sleeve for much of the time. Once the oedema is established the progressive fibrosis makes lymphoedema very much more difficult to treat.

TREATMENT

There are three main goals in the treatment of patients with no evidence of active cancer.

1. To reduce the volume and restore the shape of the affected arm to as close to the contralateral normal arm as possible.
2. To maintain the improvement in shape and size long-term.
3. To prevent acute inflammatory episodes.

To achieve these aims the treatment consists of several components, which work together to provide the right environment and the right sort of stimulus for maximum lymph drainage.

Diruetics are of limited value in the treatment of lymphoedema. They may, however, be a helpful adjunct to treatment in instances where the oedema is of mixed origin or is exacerbated by fluid-retaining drugs.

Pneumatic compression pumps are often the first line of treatment offered to patients with lymphoedema. These pumps come in a variety of models, ranging from the use of single chamber to sequential, multichambered sleeves. They all work on the same basic principle: a motor-driven pump is attached by tubing to an inflatable sleeve, into which the arm is inserted. Air is pumped into the sleeve causing it to inflate and deflate in a cycle, thereby squeezing water out of the limb.

In an oedema where the main problem is simply an excessive amount of water in the affected tissues (e.g. in a dependent or immobile limb, or in venous hypertension), pneumatic compression pumps can be extremely effective. They are capable of shifting large quantities of water out of the limb via the venous system or through tissue planes.

In lymphoedema, however, the main problem is one of protein removal. The lymphatics are the only escape route for large proteins and if they are not able to perform this function the concentration of protein in the tissues rises and osmotic forces attract more water into the tissues. The use of pumps in lymphoedema may result in a significant short-term reduction in limb volume, but unless other treatments are used to stimulate lymphatic function (and hence protein removal), the fluid simply returns and satisfactory long-term control will remain elusive.

A further word of caution: if oedema involves the root of the limb (i.e. the shoulder and axillary area) or the adjacent quadrant of the trunk, the use of a compression pump on the arm runs the risk of increasing congestion in these areas, inhibiting drainage from the arm still further.

There are four main principles of treatment (Foldi, Foldi and Weissleder, 1985):

- care of the skin;
- external support;
- movement and positioning of the limb;
- massage.

Skin care

The recurrent inflammatory episodes that are such a feature of lymphoedema lead to an acute exacerbation of swelling at the time of the attack and, if not controlled, can damage remaining lymphatic vessels through scarring of the vessel walls. Educating the patient in the prevention of infection will help reduce the risk of such attacks; this involves common sense measures such as the use of gloves when gardening or doing rough house-work, protecting the arm from heat and sunburn, and maintaining intact, supple skin. Promoting lymph drainage will also lead to the prevention of acute inflammatory episodes.

At the onset of an attack the patient often feels very unwell, with flu-like symptoms, a raised temperature and occasionally rigors. The arm may appear reddened or there may be a blotchy rash; it usually feels rather hot and tender. During an attack the emphasis is on rest and elevation (to the horizontal) of the affected arm and oral antibiotics. Treatment of the oedema should be postponed until the inflammation has subsided. Long-term prophylactic penicillin V should be considered in patients experiencing frequent, recurrent episodes of inflammation.

External support

External support on the arm is an essential component of treatment for several reasons. By applying sufficient pressure to the limb in an even pressure gradient (high distally and low proximally), fluid is encouraged to drain via the root of the limb. The pressure also helps to limit the formation of lymph by blood capillary filtration. The two main forms of support – low-stretch bandages and elastic compression sleeves – each have a distinct function and are used at a specific stage of treatment.

Bandages are used to reduce significant oedema and restore normal shape to the limb. During the reduction phase the patient is treated on a daily basis by a therapist for a course of treatment lasting between two and three weeks, depending on progress. The application of evenly graduated compression requires a certain amount of skill to avoid constriction or trauma to the limb. The bandages are applied to give high pressures over a system of padding that takes into account the shape of the limb (Badger and Twycross, 1988).

The bandages remain in place over 24 hours and are then re-applied; the padding needs to be reviewed and adjusted on a daily basis to keep pace with any change in the shape of the arm. It is not realistic to expect patients or their relatives to be able to carry out this phase of treatment themselves. While the bandages are rather bulky they should **never** cause pain or discomfort, nor should they ever result in trauma to the skin. Most patients accommodate to the unfamiliar feeling of pressure within the first 24 hours, but should be instructed to remove the bandages if they cause pain or if symptoms of impaired circulation develop.

The role of the compression sleeve, on the other hand, is to support the drained tissues and maintain limb shape and size long-term. 'Off-the-shelf' sleeves are available in a wide range of sizes and designs and are usually considerably cheaper than made-to-measure. They are not available on GP prescription but can be supplied by any hospital appliance officer.

A sleeve should always feel comfortable to wear and time and care should be taken to find the best one for each patient; an ill-fitting or uncomfortable sleeve will result in poor compliance and poor control of the oedema. When deciding on the design of sleeve, account must be taken of the extent of the oedema. It is useless to fit a patient with a sleeve that stops at the wrist if the patient has hand swelling. A patient may well have to begin by wearing a compression glove to control finger swelling together with a sleeve with integral handpiece to control hand and arm swelling. However, good compliance in the initial months of treatment will usually result in the patient gradually being able to leave off the glove and eventually the handpiece. Whether off-the-shelf or made-to-measure, hosiery needs replacing every three to four months.

At this stage of treatment the patients essentially treat themselves, the therapist providing regular follow-up and monitoring of progress together with support and encouragement. Most patients will need to wear a sleeve for several years if not for the rest of their lives.

Movement and positioning

Movement provides the main stimulus for lymph flow and the effect is enhanced if combined with support on the limb (Leduc, Peeters and Bourgeois, 1990, Olszewski and Engeset, 1990). A balance must be struck between moving the arm sufficiently to prevent pooling of fluid in the tissues, and avoiding excessive strain on the arm (e.g. lifting, carrying, pulling or pushing heavy objects) or vigorous exercise, which would result in an increase in blood flow and hence an increase in fluid formation. Positioning the arm correctly when at rest (i.e. to the horizontal) to counter the effects of gravity, will also help to maintain good lymph flow. It is not necessary to elevate the limb any higher than this, resting the arm on a pillow or cushion along the arm of a chair is sufficient.

Holding the arm across the body for long periods or flexed at the elbow usually results in pooling of fluid around the elbow and should be discouraged.

Massage

The right sort of gentle tissue movement, or massage, has been shown to be effective at stimulating lymph flow (Olszewski and Engeset, 1990). The aim is to encourage fluid to move from a congested area of the body, via existing alternative drainage routes, to areas of the body that are draining normally (Foldi, Foldi and Weissleder, 1985). In the case of unilateral upper limb swelling, this would be the contralateral normal quadrant of the body. This technique is particularly useful in cases where the root of the limb or quadrant of the body adjacent to the affected arm are congested, since extensive truncal swelling will further impede drainage of the arm. Massage always begins centrally, the swollen arm being treated last, so that the way ahead is always decongested first.

Minimal pressure is used when massaging, just sufficient to move the skin and tissues, since the aim is to stimulate superficial drainage and to avoid an increase in blood flow to the area. Good contact between the hand and the skin beneath is essential, and for this reason the area being massaged should be free of creams, oils or talcum powder.

ASSESSMENT

The patient with lymphoedema benefits enormously from a multidisciplinary approach to treatment. A thorough initial assessment will determine what other members of the multidisciplinary team need to be involved in the care of the patient. This should include a history of the patient's surgical and radiotherapy treatment and a history of the oedema.

Information about joint mobility and any neurological deficit in the swollen arm will be helpful when setting treatment goals, and an assessment of these is best performed by a physiotherapist.

Pain or discomfort is not unusual in lymphoedema (Badger *et al.*, 1988) but this needs careful evaluation. Patients typically complain of a feeling of tightness and heaviness in the swollen limb that is sometimes accompanied by a deep aching in the arm. These symptoms usually improve once treatment of the oedema has started. Neurological-type pains (e.g. stabbing, shooting, burning, numbness, tingling, etc.) are not, however, usually attributable to lymphoedema although they may be exacerbated by swelling), and usually have their origin in radiation fibrosis or tumour compression/invasion of the nerves. These types of pain will not neccessarily respond to treatment of the oedema and advice will need to be sought regarding appropriate drug or physiotherapy treatments.

An occupational therapy referral will establish which areas of day to day living the patient finds difficult as a result of her lymphoedema. A swollen hand, for example, may result in difficulties with fastening and unfastening clothing, holding a pen or other implements. Gross swelling or reduced shoulder mobility can interfere with a whole range of household and personal tasks.

Assessment of the degree and extent of swelling will help to determine the initial treatment approach. Limb volume can be calculated from circumference measurements taken every 4 cm along the length of the limb; the advantage of this method of measurement is that one can not only determine the total loss or gain in volume but can also see precisely where along the arm this loss or gain has occurred.

Mild, and in some cases moderate, swelling of recent onset can usually be managed simply with hosiery, advice on skin care, movement and positioning. The earlier the swelling is caught the easier it is to treat, and the attitude of waiting until problems develop is not to be encouraged.

Once lymphoedema is well-established the resulting tissue fibrosis makes swelling more difficult to influence. Resistant cases of moderate oedema and cases of gross oedema require more intensive measures, such as a course of bandaging. Some patients with severe oedema may require more than one course of bandaging over a period of, say, a year since progress is often in a step-wise fashion with improvement after bandaging followed by a plateau, followed in turn by improvement after a subsequent course of bandaging, etc.

Patient education is essential to enable them to cope with what is, after all, a chronic condition. A clear explanation about the cause of the swelling, and information about the factors that help and hinder lymph drainage, help to ensure good compliance and therefore a better treatment outcome.

Regular follow-up is as important as the initial treatment so that adjustments can be made in the light of any changes that occur in the patient's condition. Follow-up visits need only be every three to six months, depending on progress, and should include objective measurements of the patient's normal and swollen arm, re-assessment of the size and type of hosiery used and replacement of any worn-out hosiery. Advice on all other aspects of treatment, such as exercise, massage and skin care, need to be reinforced. Follow-up can be extended to every 12 months if the oedema remains stable, but arrangements must be made for the patient to receive new sleeves when needed.

FACTORS AFFECTING THE TREATMENT APPROACH

Limb shape

An arm that is distorted in shape, for example bulging at the forearm or upper arm, or with deepened skin folds at the wrist, will be difficult to treat with hosiery. An elastic sleeve would simply pull in at the narrow points of the arm or into the skin creases and emphasize the distorted shape. Bandages can be used to improve the shape of the limb. The padding layer under the bandage is arranged in such a way that the contour of the limb is evened out, resulting in a smooth profile on which to apply the compression bandage (Badger and Twycross, 1988). This ensures an even, graduated pressure gradient. Once the limb shape has improved an elastic sleeve can be fitted. Extra layers of compression or a more 'rigid' type of hosiery (i.e. where the hosiery material is less flexible) may need to be applied for the first few weeks after bandaging until the stretched tisses have tightened up. Shaped Tubigrip is useful for increasing compression and this can be used under or over the compression sleeve. Positioning the arm correctly at rest plays an important part in maintaining a good limb shape by allowing maximum drainage.

Severe oedema

Hosiery is not appropriate as a first line treatment for gross oedema. While an elastic sleeve may be able to prevent a worsening of the swelling, it will not be able to exert enough pressure on a very large limb to reduce severe swelling. Bandages are needed to apply sufficient pressure and can be used on any size of limb, however grossly swollen. If the swelling is very severe, the patient may require more than one course of bandaging. Once the arm is a satisfactory shape and size a compression sleeve can be fitted.

Lymphorrhoea

Leakage of lymph (lymphorrhoea) occurs when there is a break in the skin and the pressure in the tissues is such that lymph pours out through it. This may happen as a result of accidental trauma to the skin, if the skin is not able to stretch quickly enough to accommodate swelling, or if acquired lymphangiomata are present. There is an increased risk of infection when this happens and it requires prompt treatment.

Lymphorroea will resolve if pressure is applied to the limb. Bandaging is the most effective method of treatment. Ensure that the leaking area is clean and apply paraffin gauze under a thick sterile pad to prevent it adhering (the pad will absorb the leaking lymph), then bandage in the usual way. Change the wet bandages as often as necessary and maintain the pressure on the limb around the clock. The leakage usually resolves within 24 to 48 hours. Once it has resolved some sort of compression sleeve will need to be applied to control the swelling and prevent further leakage.

Fragile or damaged skin

In acute swelling the skin is often taut, shiny and fragile. In these situations pulling a well-fitting compression sleeve on and off may well cause trauma to the skin. Similarly, the skin may be liable to trauma where there are tumour metastases in the skin of the swollen arm. Bandages can be used over appropriate dressings until the condition of the skin has improved sufficiently for a compression sleeve to be fitted.

FACTORS AFFECTING TREATMENT OUTCOME

Tumour recurrence

Local tumour recurrence will obstruct lymph drainage in its area, particularly in the important lymph collaterals. If the tumour responds to cancer treatment there should be a corresponding improvement in the oedema; conversely, if the tumour is uncontrolled and progressing it will become more and more difficult to reduce the oedema. In some patients it is possible to prevent a worsening of the oedema, but this depends largely on the extent of tumour. However, even in patients with advanced disease it is usually possible, using the same treatments outlined above, to alleviate some of the discomfort caused by the tense, hard oedema that is often associated with tumour progression (Badger, 1987; Badger and Regnard, 1989).

Obesity

There is some evidence to suggest that obesity is a predisposing factor in the development of lymphoedema (Falardeau, Poljicak and Abovjaovde, 1988). It also appears to be more difficult to reduce and control lymphoedema in obese patients. It would appear that fat is laid down preferentially in lymph-oedematous limbs and it may be that the combination of increased fat deposition and obesity makes lymphoedema more difficult to influence. A low fat diet or weight reduction may result in an improved response in these patients.

Paralysis

Movement of the swollen limb is essential to maintain good lymph flow. Where movement is diminished or absent there is little or no propulsion to lymph and the result is dependency or gravitational oedema. This type of swelling is relatively easy to treat; the oedema is usually soft and pitting in nature, and the limb will often vary considerably in size over the course of the day. If the patient already suffers from lymphoedema, the addition of dependency oedema places an added burden on the already compromised lymphatics. This does not usually complicate the reduction of swelling but unless movement improves or is restored to the limb it can make lymphoedema more difficult to control long-term.

Chronic skin conditions

If chronic skin conditions (e.g. eczema, dermatitis or psoriasis) affect the swollen limb there is often an exacerbation of oedema as a result of local inflammation. There is also the added risk of infection where the skin is broken. Effective treatment of the skin condition should result in better control of the oedema.

Difficulty with hosiery

Compression sleeves must be firm-fitting to be effective. Elderly or arthritic patients may find it difficult to put on their sleeves. On the whole, careful instruction in the correct method of applying a sleeve overcomes most of the problems of application, but for those who have great difficulty sleeve applicators are available from at least one sleeve manufacturer (Medi UK Ltd, see Appendix A).

Patients with brachial plexus damage often find it easier to put on a sleeve with a separate handpiece rather than a sleeve with an integral hand piece. Using two layers of sleeves in a size slightly bigger than you would normally fit is another option worth trying; the sleeve will be easier to apply, and wearing two layers ensures sufficient pressure is applied to the limb.

Venous obstruction

A significant number of patients with breast cancer-related lymphoedema have compromised venous flow in the affected limb (Svensson *et al.*, 1990). A thorough initial assessment of the patient with arm oedema should include looking for signs of venous obstruction in the limb. If obstruction is present the arm is typically somewhat mottled in appearance with a rather dusky colour. If obstruction is acute, the arm may appear pink and warm and the patient usually complains of pain and an acute increase in swelling. There may be obvious collateral veins on the upper arm or chest wall. Normal venous pressure can be confirmed by palpating any visible veins on the back of the hand or in the anticubital fossa and elevating the arm; the veins should collapse on elevation. If they remain raised, or if the pressure increases, this suggests venous hypertension.

If the cause of the obstruction is a thrombus then anticoagulation is usually indicated and this can be combined with wearing a sleeve or the use of bandages. As the blood clot resolves much of the increased swelling will also resolve.

If venous obstruction is due to irreversible scarring from surgery, radiotherapy or local tumour, there may be difficulties in maintaining any reduction in the size of the limb. The increased venous pressure results in more lymph being formed and, as in the case of dependency oedema, this places an additional load on the already compromised lymphatics.

Occupation

Heavy use of a swollen limb will usually result in increased swelling. Patients in jobs that entail heavy manual work will find it difficult to maintain a stable limb size. Repetitive movements where the arm is fairly static, such as typing or operating certain types of machinery, can also lead to an increase in swelling. Patients who find themselves in these situations should be advised to break the movement pattern every so often and exercise the arm so that the muscles contract and relax, activating the muscle pump.

CONCLUSION

Patients with arm lymphoedema are often left to cope with the condition as best they can, with very little in the way of accurate information and advice. This is unfortunate since treatments exist to reduce swelling and, when this is not possible because of advancing disease, much can be done to alleviate discomfort. It is true to say that there is almost always something that can be done for any patient at any stage of her disease. By catching patients at an early stage, when the swelling first appears, there is every possibility that we can prevent the grossly swollen arms that prove so uncomfortable and disabling to so many breast cancer patients.

REFERENCES

Badger, C. (1987) Lymphoedema: management of patients with advanced cancer. *Professional Nurse*, **2**(4), 100–102.

Badger, C. and Regnard, C. (1989) Oedema in advanced disease: a flow diagram. *Palliative Medicine*, **3**, 213–15.

Badger, C. and Twycross, R. (1988) The Management of Lymphoedema – Guidelines. Sobell Study Centre, Oxford.

Badger, C., Mortimer, P., Regnard, C. and Twycross, R. (1988) Pain in the Chronically Swollen Limb, in *Progress in Lymphology – XI, Excerpta Medica* (Ed. H. Partsch), Elsevier, Amsterdam, pp. 243–5.

Falardeau, M., Poljicak, M. and Abovjaovde, M. (1988) Lymphoedema After Treatment of Breast Cancer, in *Progress in Lymphology – XI, Excerpta Medica* (ed. H. Partsch), pp. 289–92.

Foldi, E., Foldi, M. and Weissleder, H. (1985) Conservative treatment of lymphoedema of the limbs. *Angiology*, **36**, 171–80.

Kissen, M.W., Querci della Rovere, G., Easton, D. and Westbury, G. (1986) Risk of lymphoedema following the treatment of breast cancer. *British Journal of Surgery*, **73**, 580–4.

Leduc, O., Peeters, A. and Bourgeois, P. (1990) Bandages: Scintigraphic Demonstration of its Efficacy on Colloidal Protein Reabsorbtion During Muscle Activity. *Progress in Lymphology – XII, Excerpta Medica* (eds M. Nishi, S. Uchino and S. Yabuki), Elsevier, Tokyo, 421–3.

Mortimer, P.S. (1990) Investigation and management of lymphoedema. *Vascular Medicine Review*, **1**, 1–20.

Olszewski, W. and Engeset, A. (1990) Peripheral Lymph Dynamics, in *Progress in Lymphology – XII, Excerpta Medica* (Eds M. Nischi, S. Uchino and S. Yabuki), pp. 213–14.

Svensson, W., Al Murrani, B., Badger, C. *et al.* (1990) Colour Doppler demonstrates the venous abnormality in postradiotherapy elephantiasis chirurgica. *Clinical Radiology*, **42**(5), 382.

Sexuality and breast cancer | 15

Annie Topping

Sexuality is a term that is frequently used and often defined (some might even say ill-defined), and it is something that pervades our beliefs, prejudices, personal relationships, body image and self-esteem. This chapter aims to explore the concept of sexuality, drawing on theories or perspectives that help to explain it, with the intention of shedding some light on why an understanding or appreciation of the subject can assist us in caring for individuals living with breast cancer.

Human sexuality has been the subject of art, literature, ethics, legislation, taboo and discussion throughout the ages but it has only recently – within the last 100 years or so – become an area of consideration and concern for health care professionals. Some critics of medicine suggest that this 19th and 20th century discourse has produced the medicalization of sexuality, resulting in classification and labelling of 'abnormality', and creating a state of illness about something that is socially acquired and constructed. An example of this phenomenon is the American Psychiatric Association's *Diagnostic and Statistical Manual of Mental Disorders*, which included homosexuality as a mental disorder until 1980 (Schulman and Hammer, 1988).

In 1975 the World Health Organization defined human sexual health as:

The integration of the somatic, emotional, intellectual, and social aspects in ways that are positively enriching, and that enhance personality, communication, and love.

From this definition one can see that human sexuality and, more particularly, sexual health are all pervading. They are important aspects of life, relationships, roles, our image of ourselves and, possibly most importantly, contribute significantly to quality of life. However, it is worth emphasizing that sexuality is broader and more embracing than sexual functioning. As Mitchell (1974) succinctly states: '. . . the important point is that sexuality is a lived experience'.

Woods (1984) defined sexuality as:

> . . . a highly complex phenomenon . . . pervades human beings, influenc-
> ing their self images and feelings. It influences their relationships with
> others. In addition, sexuality involves the biologic basis for experienc-
> ing sexual pleasure, giving and receiving sensual pleasure, and is a
> powerful influence in a person's ability to bond to another person.

However, what neither of these definitions address is that human sexuality
is not a fixed entity but ever changing in response to developmental processes,
interaction with others and time; it can be affected by the experience of ill health
and, in this context, the diagnosis, treatment and adaptation to breast cancer.

Various perspectives have increased our understanding of sexuality and the
implications of illness to sexual health. These will be discussed along with
approaches the clinician can use to help clients through the experience of breast
cancer. With this goal in mind, it should be remembered that our understanding
to date is tentative and the strategies suggested are not hewn in tablets of stone.
Secondly, greater understanding and knowledge will only be achieved if we
try to appreciate the effects of breast cancer through the experiences of clients
and their important others; we should utilize their realities to enhance our
understanding.

SEXUALITY, SOCIETY AND CULTURE

Contradictions abound concerning sexuality. In the Christian tradition, women
could be said to be divided between being a madonna, or a temptress and a
whore (Weinberg, 1982). Just as homosexuality was categorized as perverse
until fairly recently, some writers see female sexuality subjugated by an
imbalance of power between men and women (De Beauvoir, 1972; Mitchell,
1974; Kelly, 1972).

Possibly the most influential figure in the field of sexuality was Sigmund
Freud. Through psychoanalytical interviews with clients, Freud built up a theory
based on anatomical differences between the sexes and the development of
distinct personalities (Webb, 1985). Freud saw early childhood as being pre-
divided between the sexes, but proposed that sensual and sexual pleasure was
gained from many body areas. On realizing that he or she has or does not have
a penis, the child becomes involved in an intra-psychic battle. The female,
feeling 'castrated' by her mother, seeks emotional attachment with the father,
thus creating her mother as a sexual rival. Resolution of this turmoil usually
occurs in puberty when the female accepts the passive nature of her sexuality
in preparation for reproductive sex.

On recognizing the importance of his penis, a boy develops fantasies about
a sexual relationship with his mother. He fears retribution from his father, who
may take away his penis, yet realizes penetration and impregnation are

the aims of sexuality. Therefore the male transfers his pleasure to the penis, thereby repressing bisexuality. Freud called these developmental processes 'Oedipal phase' (Chodorow, 1978).

Although Freud's work has been heavily criticized for various reasons – lack of scientific validity, small sample, biased sample in that his patients were the basis of the interpretation and therefore could be said to present an 'abnormal' picture – Freud's work has become influential and possibly incorporated into everyday ideas. Another aspect of Freud's influence is the development of psychoanalysis as a means of helping people with emotional difficulties, although again this technique has its critics (Brown, 1973).

Human sexual behaviour, breast cancer and relationships

Human sexual behaviour is highly variable and it is difficult to make judgements about what is normal or dysfunctional. Since the 1930s there has been a more systematic study of sexual behaviour, beginning with Kinsey *et al.* in 1948 and 1953. Although there are concerns about the reliability of the data as the respondents may have been inaccurate or creative with the truth, and the sampling may have been biased, some inferences can be drawn. Men reported more sexual activity than women at all ages, and female sexuality peaked in the 30–45 age group. Marriage was an important factor influencing frequency of sexual activity, but it was also influenced by age and length of relationship (Cole, 1988). Possibly the most influential aspect of the work of the Kinsey Institute was the explosion of myths about homosexuality, masturbation, and female orgasm.

The impact of breast cancer on relationships can be considerable. Both the woman with the disease and her partner can experience temporary or permanent sexual difficulties. The study by Wellish, Jamison and Pasnau (1978) suggested that when the man was involved in the decision-making process along with the woman they rated higher levels of sexual satisfaction before and after treatment. Although frequency of sexual activity was diminished, sexual satisfaction and frequency were correlated. This study also elicited that a man's failure to see his partner naked was often of their own choosing. Another study (Leiber *et al.*, 1976) suggested that although 25% reported a decreased desire for sexual intercourse post-treatment, 44% reported an increased desire for non-sexual physical closeness.

More recent studies exploring husbands' adjustment to breast cancer (Northouse and Swain, 1987; Northouse, 1988, 1989) have identified some interesting findings. Husbands perceived significantly less support from health care professionals than their partners throughout the course of the illness. Both wives and husbands who received support immediately around surgery reported fewer adjustment problems. The results also showed that there was a degree of mutual support. Although this study did not focus on sexual functioning, it has some value in adding to our understanding of the psychological aspects in a broader context.

Wellisch (1985) describes a number of factors that influence the impact of breast cancer on a marital relationship:

- the status of the relationship before cancer developed;
- the length of the marriage;
- the stage of the disease and the associated management ramifications;
- the point in the course of the disease;
- the interpersonal skills of the partners.

The final factor in particular has implications for the two parties in terms of their potential willingness to talk through difficulties of an especially sensitive and private nature, and it raises issues to do with the ability of the husband and wife to make use of support services.

Table 15.1 The human sexual response cycle*

	Women	Men
Excitement	Nipple erection Engorgement of breasts Increased venous dilation Clitoris enlargement Vaginal lubrication Extension and enlargement of vagina	Nipple erection Penile erection
Plateau	Increasing engorgement of primary and secondary sex organs Generalized muscle tension Hyperventilation > Heart rate Skin flush	Corpus spongiosum engorges Penile bulb enlarges Generalized muscle tension Hyperventilation > Heart rate Skin flush
Orgasm	Rhythmic contractions of the circumvaginal muscles Other muscles may have involuntary spasms Hyperventilation > Heart rate > Blood pressure	Rhythmic contractions along length of penile urethra Semen expelled Involuntary muscle spasm Hyperventilation > Heart rate > Blood pressure
Resolution	Breast and nipples return to normal size Skin rash disappears Muscle tension dissipates Respiratory rate returns to normal Relaxation of circumvaginal muscles	Nipples return to normal Penile shaft rapidly reduces in size – complete detumescence over time Respiratory rate reduces Muscle tension dissipates

Women may have multiple orgasms without returning to plateau or remaining in the resolution phase before they can be restimulated to orgasm. Most men spend a period in resolution before they can be restimulated to resolution.

*Adapted from Siemans and Bradzel (1982), Webb (1985) and Lamb (1992).

HUMAN SEXUAL RESPONSE CYCLE

Masters and Johnson (1966) conducted extensive laboratory examination of male and female sexual arousal and orgasm and found little significant difference between men and women. Table 15.1 shows a summary of the physiological changes that occur during sexual intercourse.

Experts in this area propose that dysfunction occurs in the areas of desire (drive, interest or appetite), arousal (excitement) and orgasm (Woods, 1990; Cole and Dryden, 1988). Table 15.2 describes some of the effects of treatment that may influence dysfunction in these areas.

Impaired sexual desire may or may not be a problem. Difficulties may only emerge as a result of the dissatisfaction of one partner or when behaviour falls short of an individual's expectations of him or herself. Loss of interest in sex and reduced perception of sexual arousal and satisfaction often occur in association with depression (Riley and Riley, 1988). Depression is an often-reported sequela of breast cancer and therefore careful assessment, explanation and, if appropriate, referral may help to resolve difficulties in this area.

Table 15.2 Sexual dysfunction following treatment for breast cancer: causes and symptoms

Dysfunction	Cause(s)	Symptoms
Drive	Post-operative depression/anxiety	Triedness, insomnia, constipation irritability, lethargy, withdrawal inability to show strong emotions etc.
	Effects of radiotherapy	Nausea, fatigue
	Effects of chemotherapy	Nausea, fatigue
	Effects of hormonal manipulation	Hot flushes, sweats, weight gain headaches, fatigue, light headedness, intermenstrual or post-menopausal bleeding
Arousal	Effects of radiotherapy	Skin soreness, coughing
	Effects of surgery	Pain around incision and arm on affected side
	Effects of chemotherapy	Vaginal dryness
	Effects of hormone manipulation	Vaginal dryness, increased sweating
Orgasm	Potentially all treatments could influence an individual's ability to experience orgasm because of the interplay between the psychological meaning of the disease and treatment and the physical side-effects.	

BODY IMAGE

> Breasts are exalted as the epitome of all that is most feminine and
> desirable in a woman.
>
> *Faulder, 1979*

In Western culture the breast represents more than a provider of nourishment for babies: a wander through any art gallery gives some indication of
how the breast has come to be portrayed as a symbol of femininity; similarly,
the significance of the breast as a sexual symbol cannot be ignored and is
reinforced daily in the British tabloid press; fashion through the ages has
emphasized what the breast symbolizes. It is therefore not surprising that the
diagnosis and treatment of breast cancer carries implications of threat, disfigurement and loss of intactness, and hits at the root of an individual's construc-
tion of her sexuality.

One of the most widely held assumptions about breast cancer is that its
treatment, particularly mastectomy, has profound negative effects on a woman's
body image. Although this belief should not be negated, it must be remembered
that this is not the case for all women living with breast cancer. Many women,
over a period of time, adapt to the surgery and continue to have fulfilling
lives and relationships. However, it is useful to have an understanding of
the theory underpinning the concept of body image in order to appreciate
how adaptation may or may not occur.

Body image can be described as a mental construct or picture that develops
from infancy as a result of sensory and motor development and exploration
of the world around the individual (Schilder, 1935). It is suggested that this
picture is constructed from one's perception or awareness of the size,
function and sensation of different parts of the body and, furthermore, that
individuals make investments in various parts of the body, which can be
influenced by environmental, interpersonal and temporal factors (Schilder,
1935). Fisher (1968, 1970, 1973) suggests that body image has several
elements: body boundary, body awareness and the meanings an individual
places on the various parts.

As individuals develop this mental picture, they also integrate and reassess
the value they place on constituent parts into the whole. Certain parts may
be perceived as dirty, or not to be touched by others; other parts may be considered valuable and worthy of enhancement by posture, clothing, make-up,
etc. The valuing of body parts may change with age and can be different from
one person to another, and from culture to culture. Some writers suggest that
body image is separate from, but can be influenced by, sexuality, whereas
others see sexuality and body image as inseparable; this latter view is adopted
in this chapter.

To aid discussion, body image will be divided into the three aspects proposed
by Price (1990).

- Body reality – as it exists, genetic make-up, wear and tear of life, 'warts and all'.
- Body ideal – the mental picture of how we would like to look; this is influenced by societal and cultural norms and threatened by changes in body reality.
- Body presentation – how we present to the outside world: how we dress, walk, pose, utilize 'props', etc; it is laden with symbolic value.

The way individuals integrate or balance these three aspects of the whole is dynamic and thus undergoing constant change and redefinition. Within the context of breast cancer, the theory can be applied as follows: the discovery of a breast lump may cause disequilibrium in body reality and reinforce dissonance with body ideal, thereby producing altered behaviour in terms of body presentation and an unhealthy total body image.

For example: a woman who has just undergone simple mastectomy is forced, by the surgery, to reconstruct her body reality to include this change. Her body ideal is intactness of breasts and this is constantly reinforced by the media, advertising, 'normal' women, etc. She may demonstrate it by refusing to get dressed in outdoor clothing, to go out of the home, to allow her partner to see the scar or her naked body, or by refusing to resume her previous sexual relationship. In sociological terms she perceives herself as abnormal (or stigmatized), she demonstrates this in her behaviour, and it is reinforced in her interactions with others (Goffman, 1968).

The example used is an extreme but serves to demonstrate the relationship between aspects of body image and the whole. Body image is also related to self-concept, self-esteem and personal identity; self-concept is another aspect of an individual's mental picture representing his or her construct of self.

It is suggested that self-concept is also made up of various elements: the body self – body image; interpersonal self – interactions with others; achieving self – aspirations and goals; and identification self – values, beliefs and prejudices (Schain and Howards, 1985). Self-concept and personal identity are often considered interchangeable, although Tabachnick (1967) views them as separate: personal identity being a combination of relationships with the outside world, and personal autonomy being reflected in a person's ability to balance the two. Self-esteem is the total value of all these concepts which together make up personal worth, so a loss of or change to, any of these aspects may result in a devaluing of self or reduced self-esteem.

Although there is some disagreement among writers about what makes up body image, self-concept and self-esteem, what does not appear to be in dispute is the correlation between poor self-esteem and negative body-image. Possibly more importantly, there is a correlation between altered body image, poor self-esteem and psychological morbidity (depression and anxiety states) in individuals with breast cancer (Jamison, Wellisch and Pasnau, 1978; Maguire *et al.*, 1980a, 1980b; Watson *et al.*, 1988).

RESEARCH RELATED TO BREAST CANCER AND SEXUALITY

Exploration of the pscyhological and sexual implications of the diagnosis and treatment of breast cancer has increased our insight into the multidimensional aspects of individuals' responses to this disease. (This chapter concentrates on the theme of sexuality and should be read in conjunction with Chapter 2.) The literature gives the clinician some understanding of the difficulties faced by many individuals, but the reality of living with breast cancer has not yet been fully explored.

In a two-year follow-up study of women who had undergone mastectomy, Morris, Greer and White (1977) reported minimal effects on marital adjustment, although 32% of respondents described deterioration of sexual functioning within the period. This study also found that poor sexual adjustment at three months post-surgery was associated with less likelihood of a return to pre-operative levels of sexual functioning at two years. The control group in this study also reported similar levels of deterioration and this was thought to be explained by the pre-menopausal status of the sample.

Early work concentrated predominantly on the effects of mastectomy on sexuality; however, current evidence suggests that for some women with breast cancer conservative treatment, or lumpectomy with or without radiotherapy, may be an equally effective treatment and could have fewer implications for sexual functioning. Fallowfield *et al.* (1990) reviewed 13 studies which compared the psychological impact of mastectomy with that of lumpectomy, and found that none identified a significant difference between the two treatments in terms of depression and anxiety, although:

> . . . most studies reported a reduction in problems relating to body image in women who did not lose a breast . . . this advantage was offset by greater fears of cancer and its possible recurrence.

Ashcroft, Leinster and Slade (1985) conducted a small study in which, where possible, women were offered a choice between mastectomy, lumpectomy or radiotherapy. Their results indicate that the importance an individual attaches to her appearance could be an important factor in her decision-making on treatment options, and that the value a woman places on maintaining a complete body image pre-operatively, when given a choice of treatment, may positively influence the psychological outcome.

Fallowfield *et al.* (1990) conducted a retrospective study of women aged less than 70 with early breast cancer who were randomly assigned to breast conservation or mastectomy. They found that over a third of women in both groups reported a loss of interest in sex since diagnosis and treatment.

A small study conducted by Maguire *et al.* (1980a) compared women undergoing mastectomy with a group that had mastectomy and adjuvant chemotherapy. Of this latter group (given cyclophosphamide, methotrexate, and 5-fluorouracil (CMF)), 70% experienced a severe loss of interest in sex following treatment.

Another aspect of the management of breast cancer is related to the issue of breast reconstruction. Schain *et al.* (1985) describe the position most eloquently:

> The major concern today is not so much whether to reconstruct a particular patient's breast but when in the sequence of treatment or rehabilitation is the best time.

In studies evaluating the psychological adjustment of mastectomy patients who had immediate reconstruction compared with those whose reconstruction was delayed, the results would appear to favour sooner rather than later (Schain *et al.*, 1985; Stevens *et al.*, 1984). As a result of their retrospective study , Schain *et al.* (1985) support the view that an externally worn prosthesis is never fully integrated into a woman's body image; in their study 39% of women gave a desire to improve sexual relations, and 19% gave a desire to change marital status, as reasons for wanting breast reconstruction. The authors warn that breast reconstruction is not necessarily a remedy for an unsuccessful marriage or relationship. In a small prospective study Stevens *et al.* (1984) came to the conclusion that immediate breast reconstruction was accompanied by a lower incidence of psychological distress post-operatively. However, these findings should be viewed with reservation. Both studies used small unrepresentative samples and were conducted in the USA. Further work needs to be done in this area before it can be suggested that early reconstruction should be routinely offered to women.

In summary, this review of the literature suggests:

1. Mastectomy as a treatment option carries the likelihood of psychological implications and/or sexual problems for a proportion of women. The chances of this are possibly greater for individuals who invest highly in an intact body image and who may therefore experience body image disturbance.
2. Conservation treatment without choice carries a similar risk of development of psychological morbidity, depression, anxiety and sexual difficulties. These are less likely to be related to body image disturbance.
3. Patient choice, based on an understanding of the options and supported decision-making, **may** reduce psychological morbidity and sexual difficulties.
4. Women undergoing adjuvant therapy appear to experience high levels of sexual disinterest.
5. Early reconstruction (for suitable candidates) may possibly reduce psychological impact, particularly in relation to body image integrity and sexual functioning.

Unfortunately, the majority of the literature exploring the emotional ramifications of breast cancer has not focused exclusively on sexual functioning, nor has it addressed other aspects of sexuality such as gender, body image, the interface between the level of ill health and/or disability and sexual behaviour as an integrated whole (Bransfield, 1982/83). The literature has also not considered the different responses to the disease among women of different ethnic backgrounds, classes or sexual proclivities. It could therefore be suggested that there is plenty of scope for researchers to continue to explore the lived experience of breast cancer and its effects on sexuality.

APPROACHES FOR ADDRESSING SEXUALITY WITH CLIENTS

It cannot be stressed too much that in discussing sexuality with a client one is asking her to disclose something that is personal and private. The trust she thus places in the clinician should not be minimized or abused, and she should be treated in a non-judgemental way with sensitivity, tact and care.

The literature suggests a number of different approaches for communicating effectively with clients and their partners about sexuality (Annon, 1974; MacElveen-Hoehn, 1985; Schover and Jensen, 1986; Webb, 1985). One approach that is widely advocated is Annon's PLISSIT model, P-LI-SS-IT being an acronym for Permission, Limited Information, Specific Suggestions, and Intensive Therapy.

Permission is the first level and encourages the client to discuss the impact of cancer and its treatment within the context of her prior and desired sexual experience. At its most basic it is giving clients the cue that it is all right to want to be sexual, that it is fine to talk about any aspect of sexuality, and that the clinician wants to help. Some individuals may not wish to talk about this part of their lives, but, if the subject is introduced appropriately it will not be perceived as threatening, and the seeds will have been sewn so that a client knows she can come back to you for a discussion if she changes her mind.

Limited information involves assessing clients' real concerns and providing them with the appropriate information or guidance. Their fear may be reduced by the offering of relevant information and support.

Specific suggestions is a level of intervention that requires more than an invitation to talk or specific information. In relation to cancer this level usually focuses on a couple's ability to communicate with each other, their physical intimacy, options for sexual expression, changing behaviours and symptom management. This level of intervention often involves a planned approach with follow-up sessions to explore progress.

Intensive therapy is the stage at which the couple or client is referred to a therapist – e.g. clinical psychologist, sexual therapist, social worker, psychiatrist, nurse specialist – with whom medical information is shared.

This level of approach is necessary when a couple's relationship is stressed or when an individual is experiencing severe difficulties. Commitment and a willingness to change is an important part of this level of intervention.

Annon (1974) claims that if permission is given a large proportion of difficulties can be resolved at that level. Clinicians working in this area with clients should be aware of their own limitations and refer to a specialist before embarking on a level of intervention beyond their skills.

SPECIFIC SEXUAL DIFFICULTIES ASSOCIATED WITH THE MANAGEMENT OF BREAST CANCER

Once the importance of considering sexuality as a vital aspect of the whole management of the patient has been understood, the clinician faced with a client with a specific difficulty will want to know how best to help. The remainder of this chapter focuses on specific problems, strategies and information. It should be remembered that matters to do with sex are personal and private and should be dealt with in a sensitive manner.

Routine screening

Women invited for breast screening know there is a chance that the investigation will show they have breast cancer, and they may therefore feel threatened by the procedure. For a tiny proportion of women this will be their introduction to living with breast cancer. It could be proposed that even at this stage empathetic support and listening are valuable along with appropriate information-giving. Although the psychological ramifications of routine screening have not yet been established, it is potentially a point of uncertainty and some clients may wish to explore this.

Diagnosis

If a woman has discovered a breast lump, sought advice and now been diagnosed as having breast cancer, she is probably in a state of shock. Although the research reviewed earlier suggests that treatment choice may have an influence on later psychosexual adaptation, the individual is probably still trying to deal with the actual diagnosis, so that discussion of options and initial assessments needs to be supportive, informative, and empathetic.

It is appropriate to introduce the subject of sexuality at this point for a number of reasons. Firstly, if the individual has the opportunity to choose between treatment options her decision should be informed. Secondly, in order to make an informed decision the client may wish to talk through the implications of specific treatments on body image and attempt to anticipate what the various options may mean in terms of her sexuality and subsequent sexual activity. Thirdly, discussing sexuality in an open way puts it firmly on the agenda, giving the client the understanding that she is able to discuss this aspect of herself. Finally, obtaining baseline information may help the assessment process preliminary to individualized care.

Surgery

On being admitted for surgery and immediately post-operatively, the first realization of what is happening may only just be dawning on the client. If she has undergone lumpectomy or mastectomy she will have a scar and some change to the prior appearance of the breast. However minimal the change, it has to be reintegrated into the whole body reality. It has been suggested that a scar can serve as a constant reminder of the wholeness lost.

Obviously, following mastectomy or wedge resection the change in terms of cosmetic appearance of the breast is greater. A number of authors suggest that a readiness to look at the scar is an important part of the process of reintegrating change into the whole (Lamb, 1992; Denton, 1989; Riley and Riley, 1988), but how this is managed is important. Whether this occurs in hospital prior to discharge or at home it is necessary to prepare the individual. These preparations may include discussion and actual drawings of what to expect, privacy and uninterrupted time, a mirror to help visualization, and allowing the individual to decide when she wishes to look. Some women may choose to have their partners with them, and this should be explored. Opportunity to reflect is also valuable.

Fear of rejection or actual rejection following breast surgery is a frequent concern. The concerns of a woman who does not have a sexual partner may focus on unacceptability, her own reluctance to establish relationships, and how to manage initiating a sexual relationship. The concerns of women within an established relationship may be real or imagined. Encouragement to resume her previous behaviour and levels of modesty is the ideal. However, some women may wish to discuss ways of reducing the confrontation of their partner with their changed image. Suggestions may include wearing nightclothes that allow a prosthesis to be worn, e.g. a night bra, and if breast stimulation is part of her normal foreplay, the woman may wish to wear a breast-feeding bra that allows the breast to be exposed while retaining the prosthesis in place. Other strategies include undressing before the partner does, sexual intercourse in the dark, and alternative positions that reduce contact with the breast or affected side.

Clients and their partners may wish to talk about the resumption of sexual activity on discharge. They may also seek advice on ways to reduce trauma or pain to the scar or affected arm. Discuss the client's usual approach to sexual expression, focusing particularly on the role of breast stimulation, positions for love-making, and her attitude (and that of her partner, if appropriate) to the loss of the breast. Another consideration is to ask the client for any ideas she may have for coping with the changes: they may be more realistic than the clinician's!

With the baseline information provided earlier it will be easier to give suggestions and tailor information according to need. Possibly the most important role the clinician can have is encouraging the client and her partner to discuss openly and honestly their feelings, hopes and attitudes in a mutually supportive way, although this is not always possible.

The following may be helpful suggestions.

Methods to reduce pain

- Relaxation techniques;
- analgesia before intercourse;
- warm bath before intercourse
- adopt a different position for intercourse.

Alternative positions

Ensure you ascertain what is acceptable.

- Male astride with pillow to protect scar;
- female astride $+/-$ pillows to support affected arm;
- side-lying with creative use of pillows to support affected arm/shoulder;
- rear entry with pillows protecting chest/arm.

Radiotherapy

Whatever the method of delivery, direct beam or interstitial, some individuals experience skin reactions. These can range from slight redness to moist desquamation. Close physical contact with the affected areas can be reduced by using alternative positions for love-making.

Radiotherapy can also cause a general lethargy and clients should be warned that their desire for sexual intercourse may therefore be reduced. Talking to clients about when they have most energy during the day and giving permission to experiment may prove helpful both during and following treatment.

Chemotherapy

Feelings of exhaustion and a reduction in libido may also result from chemotherapy. Most protocols are delivered in a cyclical fashion, so encouraging clients to monitor when they have most energy may help them to identify the best times for sexual activity. As most regimes induce a degree of immunosuppression, information should be given on reducing the risk of developing opportunistic infections such as candida. The use of condoms for protection should be encouraged.

Pre-menopausal clients should be informed that their menstrual cycle may be affected and may take a variable length of time to return to normal. Methods of preventing pregnancy during treatment and for at least 12 months afterwards should be discussed.

Some women experience menopausal symptoms during chemotherapy, which can be disconcerting. Reduced vaginal secretions may make sexual intercourse painful: the use of water soluble lubricants or saliva may help to reduce discomfort, and extended foreplay may help to increase the natural production of secretions. Clients should be discouraged from douching as this disrupts normal flora and increases dryness.

Hormone manipulation therapy

Ovarian ablation, whether surgical or as a result of radiotherapy or endocrine therapy, will produce menopausal symptoms in pre-menopausal women. As in a normally occurring menopause, symptoms such as hot sweats, reduced libido, weight gain and vaginal dryness are common. This can be particularly distressing for these women: not only have they had to face breast cancer, and possibly chemotherapy or radiotherapy, but they are now experiencing the premature onslaught of symptoms that remind them that they are no longer able to reproduce. Sensitive and supportive listening, allowing women to vocalize their fears, along with sound information and advice on symptom control may help them to cope with this event.

Post-menopausal patients may still experience symptoms of reduced libido, weight gain and increased vaginal dryness. These should be discussed and possible strategies to employ should be suggested.

CONCLUSION

Throughout the literature concerning sexuality, a recurrent theme is that health care professionals have difficulties dealing with clients in this aspect of their lives (Lief and Payne, 1975; Fisher and Levin, 1983; Webb and Askham, 1987; Wilson and Williams, 1988; Waterhouse and Metcalfe, 1991).

I hope that this chapter goes some way to providing a resource for clinicians helping clients to adapt to a disease process that has implications for their sexual health. For those embarking on new territory, I give some words of warning from Ray, Grover and Wesniewski (1984):

A cheerful and optimistic manner can discourage the expression of negative attitudes by the patient, and too great a readiness to provide reassurance may mean this is given before the nature of a patient's worries have been clarified.

The reader may have noticed that the term counselling has not been used. This was deliberate but is not intended to negate the valuable work many clinicians undertake in this area. If one looks at the many definitions associated with the word counselling, the central issue is that it is:

a process through which one person helps another by purposeful conversation in an understanding atmosphere . . . its basic purpose is to assist the individual to make their own decisions from among the choices available.

British Association of Counselling, 1969

I would consider that, unfortunately, the level of interaction of health care professionals with clients in relation to sexuality does not always fulfil that definition. I would hope that we go some way to giving clients useful information and allowing them to express their concerns. Counselling is for the trained and experienced, and in an area as sensitive as sexuality we need to tread carefully.

REFERENCES

Annon, J.S. (1974) *The behavioural treatment of sexual problems*, Mercantile Printing, Honolulu.

Ashcroft, J.J., Leinster, S.J. and Slade, P.D. (1985) Breast Cancer – Patient choice of treatment: preliminary communication. *Journal of Research Social Medicine*, **78**, 43–46.

Bransfield, D.D. (1982/3) Breast cancer and sexual functioning: a review of the literature and implications for future research. *International Journal of Psychiatry in Medicine,* **12**, 197–211.

British Association of Counselling (1969) *Steering Committee of the Standing Conference for the Advancement of Counselling*, BAC, Rugby.

Brown, P. (1973) *Radical Psychology*, Harper & Row, New York.

Chodorow, N. (1978) *The Reproduction of Mothering. Psychoanalysis and the Sociology of Gender*, University of California Press, Berkeley.

Cole, M. (1988) Normal and dysfunctional sexual behaviour, frequencies and incidencies, in *Sex Therapy in Britain* (eds M. Cole and W. Dryden), Open University Press, Milton Keynes, pp. 12–48.

Cole, M. and Dryden, W. (1988) *Sex Therapy in Britain*, Open University Press, Milton Keynes, p. 4.

de Beauvoir, S. (1972) *The Second Sex*, Penguin, Harmondsworth.

Denton, S. (1989) Nursing Patients with Breast Cancer, in *Oncology for Nurses and*

Health Care Professionals Volume III, 2nd edn (ed. D. Borley), Harper & Row, Beaconsfield, pp. 309–39.

Fallowfield, L.J., Hall, A., Maguire, G.P. and Baum, M. (1990) Psychological outcomes of different treatment policies in women with early breast cancer outside clinical trials. *British Medical Journal*, **301**(6752), 575–80.

Faulder, C. (1979) *Breast Cancer: A guide to Its Early Detection and Treatment*, Pan Books, London.

Fisher, S. (1968) *Body Image and Personality*, Dover Press, New York.

Fisher, S. (1970) *Body experience in fantasy and behaviour*, Appleton-Century-Crofts, New York.

Fisher, S. (1973) *Body Consciousness: You are what you feel*, Prentice Hall, Eaglewood Cliffs.

Fisher, S.G. and Levin, D.L. (1983) The sexual knowledge and attitudes of professional nurses caring for oncology patients. *Cancer Nursing*, **6**, 55–61.

Goffman, E. (1968) *Stigma: Notes on the Management of the Spoiled Identity*, Penguin, Harmondsworth.

Jamison, K.R., Wellisch, D.K. and Pasnau, R.O. (1978) Psychosocial aspects of mastectomy: I The Woman's Perspective. *American Journal of Psychiatry*, **133**(4), 432–6.

Kelly, J. (1972) Sister love; an exploration of the need for homosexual experience. *Family Coordinator*, October.

Kinsey, A.C., Pomeroy, W.B., Martin, C.E. and Gebherd, P.H. (1948) *Sexual Behaviour in the Human Male*, W.B. Saunders and Co., Philadelphia.

Kinsey, A.C., Pomeroy, W.B., Martin, C.E. and Gebherd, P.H. (1953) *Sexual Behaviour in the Human Female*, W.B. Saunders and Co., Philadelphia.

Lamb, M.A. (1992) Alterations in Sexuality and Sexual Functioning, in *Cancer Nursing A Comprehensive Textbook* (eds S. Baird, R. McCorkle and M. Grant), W.B. Saunders and Co., Philadelphia, 831–49.

Leiber, L., Plumb, M.M., Herstenzang, M.L. and Holland, J. (1976) The communication of affection between cancer patients and their spouses. *Psychosomatic Medicine*, **38**(6), 379–89.

Lief, H.I. and Payne, T. (1975) Sexuality – knowledge and attitudes. *American Journal of Nursing*, **75**(11), 2026–9.

MacElveen-Hoehn, P. (1985) Sexual assessment and counselling. *Seminars in Oncology Nursing*, **1**, 69–75.

Maguire, G.P., Tait, A., Brooke, M. *et al.* (1980a) Psychiatric morbidity and physical toxicity with adjuvant chemotherapy after mastectomy. *British Medical Journal*, **281**(6249), 1179–80.

Maguire, G.P., Tait, A., Brooke, M. *et al.* (1980b) Effect of counselling on the psychiatric morbidity associated with mastectomy. *British Medical Journal*, **2**, 1454–6.

Masters, W.H. and Johnson, V.E. (1966) *Human Sexual Response*, Little Brown & Co., Boston.

Mitchell, J. (1974) *Psychoanalysis and Feminism*, Penguin, Harmondsworth, p. 304.

Morris, T., Greer, S. and White, P. (1977) Psychological and social adjustment to mastectomy: a two year follow-up study. *Cancer*, **40**, 2381–7.

Northouse, L.L. (1988) Social support in patients' and husbands' adjustment to breast cancer. *Nursing Research* **37**(2), 91–5.

Northouse, L.L. (1989) A longitudinal study of the adjustment of patients and husbands to breast cancer. *Oncology Nursing Forum*, **16**(4), 511–16.

Northouse, L.L. and Swain, M.A. (1987) Adjustment of patients and husbands to the initial impact of cancer. *Nursing Research* **36**(4), 221–5.

Price, B. (1990) A model for body-image care. *Journal of Advanced Nursing* **15**(5), 585–93.

Ray, C., Grover, J. and Wesniewski, T. (1984) Nurses' perceptions of early breast cancer and mastectomy, and their psychological imiplications, and the role of health professionals in providing support. *International Journal of Nursing Studies* **21**(2), 101–11.

Riley, A.J. and Riley, E.J. (1988) Sex therapy in patients with medical problems, in *Sex Therapy in Britain* (eds M. Cole and W. Dryden), Open University Press, Milton Keynes, pp. 264–71.

Schain, W.S. and Howards, S.S. (1985) Sexual Problems of Patients with Cancer, in *Cancer: Principles and Practice of Oncology*, 2nd edn (eds V.T. De Vita Jnr, S. Hellman and S. Rosenberg), J.B. Lippincott, Phildelphia, pp. 2066–82.

Schain, W.S., Wellisch, D.K., Pasnau, R.O. and Lansverk, J. (1985) The sooner the better: a study of psychological factors in women undergoing immediate versus delayed breast reconstruction. *American Journal of Psychiatry* **142**(1), 40–6.

Schilder, P. (1935) *The image and appearance of the human body. Studies in the constructive energies of the psyche*, Kegan Paul, London.

Schover, L.R. and Jensen, S.B. (1986) *Sexuality and Chronic Illness: a comprehensive approach*, Guildford Press, New York and London.

Schulman, G.L. and Hammer, J. (1988) Social characteristics, the diagnosis of mental disorders, and the change from DSM II to DSM III. *Sociology of Health and Illness* **10**(4), 542–60.

Stevens, L.A., McGrath, M.H., Druss, R.G. *et al.* (1984) The psychological impact of immediate breast reconstruction for women with early breast cancer. *Plastic and Reconstructive Surgery*, **73**(4), 619–26.

Tabachnick, N. (1967) Self-realization and social definition: two aspects of identity formation. *International Journal of Psychoanalysis*, **48**, 68–75.

Waterhouse, J. and Metcalfe, M. (1991) Attitudes to nurses discussing sexual concerns with patients. *Journal of Advanced Nursing*, **16**(9), 1048–54.

Watson, M., Denton, S., Baum, M. and Greer, S. (1988) Counselling breast cancer patients: a specialist nursing service. *Counselling Psychology Quarterly* **1**(1), 23–32.

Webb, C. (1985) *Sexuality, Nursing and Health*, John Wiley & Sons, Chichester, p. 33.

Webb, C. and Askham, J. (1987) Nurses' knowledge and attitudes about sexuality in health care – a review of the literature. *Nurse Education Today* **7**(2), 75–87.

Wellisch, D.K. (1985) The psychological impact of breast cancer on relationships. *Seminars in Oncology Nursing*, **1**, 195–9.

Wellisch, D.K., Jamison, K.R. and Pasnau, R.O. (1978) Psychosocial Aspects of

Mastectomy: II The Man's Perspective. *American Journal of Psychiatry*, **135**(5), 543–6.

Wilson, M.E. and Williams, H.A. (1988) Oncology nurses' attitudes and behaviours related to sexuality of patients with cancer. *Oncology Nursing Forum* **15**(1) 49–53.

Woods, N.F. (1984) *Human Sexuality in Health and Illness*, C.V. Mosby, St Louis.

Woods, N.F. (1990) *Human Sexuality in Health and Illness*, 3rd edn, C.V. Mosby, St Louis.

World Health Organization (1975) *Education and Treatment in Human Sexuality: The Training of Health Professionals, Report of a WHO Meeting*, Technical Report Series No. 572, WHO, Geneva.

Appendix A: Useful addresses

Breakthrough Breast Cancer
Pauline O'Brien
PO Box 2JP
London
W1A 2JP

Breast Cancer Care (formerly Breast Care and Mastectomy Association)
Kiln House, 210 New Kings Road
London
SW6 4NZ
Tel: 0171-384 2984 (administration)
    0171-384 2344 (helpline)
    0500 245345 (freeline)

British Association of Cancer United Patients (BACUP)
3 Bath Place
Rivington Street
London
EC2A 3JR
Tel: 0171-613 2121
    0800 181199 (freephone)

Cancerlink
17 Britannia Street
London
WC1X 9JN
Tel: 0171-833 2451 and 0131-228 5557 (general enquiries)
    0800 591028 (Macline – freephone number for young people
    affected by cancer)
    0171-713 7867 (Asian Cancer Care Information – in Bengali)

Women's National Cancer Control Campaign
1 South Audley Street
London
W1Y 5DQ
Tel: 0171-729 1735 (administration)
    0171-729 2229 (helpline)
    0171-729 4915 (breast cancer information tape)

Appendix B: Companies currently supplying external silicone prostheses and mastectomy clothing

Company	Products
Amoena (UK) Ltd 18 Monks Brook Park School Close Chandlers Ford East Leigh Hampshire SO53 4RA Tel: 01703-270345	Amoena Natura Tria range Classic Classic Light Extra Soft Partial Lingerie and bras Priform Nipples Self-supporting breast forms Tinting services
Anita International Ltd Unit 6B The Foundry London Road Kingsworthy Winchester SO23 7QD Tel: 01962-883400	Anita prostheses Bras and swimwear
Breast Cancer Care Kiln House, 210 New Kings Road, London SW6 4NZ Tel: 0171-384 2984	Temporary prostheses, prostheses and information on prosthetics and clothing

CAMP Ltd
Portfield Industrial Estate
Nevil Shute Road
Portsmouth
PO3 5RC

A complete range of
   prostheses supplied
Swimwear and bras

Tel: 01 705-697411 (Portsmouth)

Medimac
15 St. Mary's House
St. Mary's Road
Shoreham-by-Sea
West Sussex
BN4S 5ZA

'Nearly Me' breast prostheses
Swim pads
Bras and swimear

Tel: 01903-816242

Medi UK Ltd
Fields Yard
Plough Lane
Hereford
HR4 0EL

Compression garments specifically
   designed for the control
   and treatment of lymphoedema

Tel: 01432-351682

Remploy Healthcare Group
Spencer Medical
Spencer House
Britannia Road
Banbury
Oxfordshire
OX16 8DP

Silima prostheses
Oval
Long oval
Heart-shaped
New assymmetrical
Bras
'Silhouette' range

Tel: 01295-275333

Trulife Ltd
9–15 Grundy Street
Liverpool
L5 95G
Tel: 0151-207 5690

Supreme range
Rhapsody
Isis
Partial prostheses
Duet adhesive
Nipples
Lecoeur

Index